ABC of
Clinical Electrocardiography
Second Edition

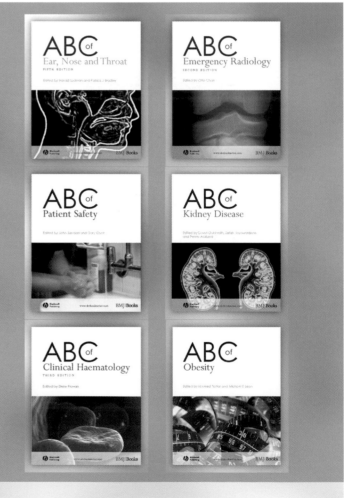

ABC of

Clinical Electrocardiography

Second Edition

Edited by

Francis Morris
Consultant in Emergency Medicine
Northern General Hospital, Sheffield

William J Brady
Professor
Department of Emergency Medicine
University of Virginia, Charlottesville, VA, USA

John Camm
Professor of Clinical Cardiology
St George's Hospital Medical School, London

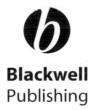

Blackwell
Publishing

BMJ|Books

© 2008 by Blackwell Publishing Ltd
BMJ Books is an imprint of the BMJ Publishing Group Limited, used under licence

Blackwell Publishing, Inc., 350 Main Street, Malden, Massachusetts 02148-5020, USA
Blackwell Publishing Ltd, 9600 Garsington Road, Oxford OX4 2DQ, UK
Blackwell Publishing Asia Pty Ltd, 550 Swanston Street, Carlton, Victoria 3053, Australia

First published 2003
Second edition 2008

1 2008

Library of Congress Cataloging-in-Publication Data

ABC of clinical electrocardiography / edited by Francis Morris, William J. Brady, John Camm. – 2nd ed.
       p. ; cm.
    Includes index.
    ISBN 978-1-4051-7064-2 (alk. paper)
    1. Electrocardiography. I. Morris, Francis. II. Brady, William, 1960- III. Camm, A. John.
 [DNLM: 1. Electrocardiography. WG 140 A134 2008]
 RC683.5.E5A23 2008
 616.1′207547–dc22

                                                     2008000428

A catalogue record for this title is available from the British Library

Set in 9.25/12 Minion by Newgen Imaging Systems Pvt Ltd, Chennai, India
Printed and bound in Singapore by COS Printers Pte Ltd

Commissioning Editor: Mary Banks
Editorial Assistant: Laura McDonald
Production Controller: Rachel Edwards

For further information on Blackwell Publishing, visit our website:
www.blackwellpublishing.com

The publisher's policy is to use permanent paper from mills that operate a sustainable forestry policy, and which has been manufactured from pulp processed using acid-free and elementary chlorine-free practices. Furthermore, the publisher ensures that the text paper and cover board used have met acceptable environmental accreditation standards.

Contents

Contributors

William J Brady
Professor,
Department of Emergency Medicine,
University of Virginia, Charlottesville, VA, USA

Kevin Channer
Consultant Cardiologist, Royall Hallamshire Hospital,
Sheffield, UK

David Da Costa
Consultant Physician, Northern General Hospital, Sheffield, UK

Daniel DeBehnke
Department of Emergency Medicine, Medical College of
Wisconsin, Milwaukee, WI, USA

June Edhouse
Consultant in Emergency Medicine, Stepping Hill Hospital,
Stockport, UK

Demas Esberger
Consultant in Accident and Emergency Medicine,
Queen's Medical Centre, Nottingham, UK

Robert French
Department of Emergency Medicine,
Medical College of Wisconsin, Milwaukee, WI, USA

Chris A Ghammaghami
Assistant Professor of Emergency and Internal Medicine,
Director, Chest Pain Centre, Department of Emergency Medicine,
University of Virginia, Charlottesville, VA, USA

Steve Goodacre
Professor of Emergency Medicine,
Medical Care Research Unit,
University of Sheffield, Sheffield, UK

Richard Harper
Assistant Professor of Emergency Medicine,
Temple University School of Medicine,
Associate Research Director, Division of Emergency Medicine,
Temple University Hospital, Philadelphia, PA, USA

Richard A Harrigan
Associate Professor of Emergency Medicine,
Department of Emergency Medicine,
Temple University School of Medicine, Philadelphia, PA, USA

Stephen Hawes
Department of Emergency Medicine, Wythenshaw Hospital,
Manchester, UK

Jonathan Hill
Specialist Registrar in Cardiology, Barts and the London NHS
Trust, London, UK

Richard Irons
Consultant in Accident and Emergency Medicine,
Princess of Wales Hospital, Bridgend, UK

Richard Jenkins
Specialist Registrar in General Medicine and Endocrinology,
Northern General Hospital, Sheffield, UK

Kevin Jones
Consultant Chest Physician, Bolton Royal Hospital, Bolton, UK

Sallyann Jones
Specialist Registrar in Accident and Emergency Medicine,
Queen's Medical Centre, Nottingham, UK

Jihad M Khalil
Thoracic and Cardiovascular Institute,
Michigan State University, Lancing, MI, USA

Jennifer H Lindsey
Fellow, Division of Cardiology, Department of Pediatrics,
University of Virginia Health System, Charlottesville, VA, USA

Karen McLeod
Consultant Paediatric Cardiologist,
Royal Hospital for Sick Children, Glasgow, UK

Steve Meek
Consultant in Emergency Medicine, Royal United Hospitals,
Bath, UK

Francis Morris
Consultant in Emergency Medicine,
Northern General Hospital, Sheffield, UK

Corey Slovis
Professor of Emergency Medicine and Medicine,
Vanderbilt University Medical Center,
Department of Emergency Medicine, Nashville, TN, USA

R K Thakur
Professor of Medicine, Thoracic and
Cardiovascular Institute, Michigan State University, Lancing,
MI, USA

Adam Timmis
Consultant Cardiologist, London Chest Hospital,
Barts and the London NHS Trust, London, UK

Preface

To my mind electrocardiogram interpretation is all about pattern recognition. This collection of 18 articles covers all the important patterns encountered in emergency medicine. Whether you are a novice or an experienced clinician, I hope that you find this book enjoyable and clinically relevant.

Francis Morris
Sheffield

CHAPTER 1

Introduction. I—Leads, Rate, Rhythm, and Cardiac Axis

Steve Meek, Francis Morris

Electrocardiography is a fundamental part of cardiovascular assessment. It is an essential tool for investigating cardiac arrhythmias and is also useful in diagnosing cardiac disorders such as myocardial infarction. Familiarity with the wide range of patterns seen in the electrocardiograms of normal subjects and an understanding of the effects of non-cardiac disorders on the trace are prerequisites to accurate interpretation.

The contraction and relaxation of cardiac muscle results from the depolarisation and repolarisation of myocardial cells. These electrical changes are recorded via electrodes placed on the limbs and chest wall and are transcribed on to graph paper to produce an electrocardiogram (commonly known as an ECG).

The sinoatrial node acts as a natural pacemaker and initiates atrial depolarisation. The impulse is propagated to the ventricles by the atrioventricular node and spreads in a coordinated fashion throughout the ventricles via the specialised conducting tissue of the His-Purkinje system. Thus, after delay in the atrioventricular node, atrial contraction is followed by rapid and coordinated contraction of the ventricles.

The electrocardiogram is recorded on to standard paper travelling at a rate of 25 mm/s. The paper is divided into large squares, each measuring 5 mm wide and equivalent to 0.2 s. Each large square is five small squares in width, and each small square is 1 mm wide and equivalent to 0.04 s.

The electrical activity detected by the electrocardiogram machine is measured in millivolts. Machines are calibrated so that a signal with an amplitude of 1 mV moves the recording stylus vertically 1 cm. Throughout this text, the amplitude of waveforms will be expressed as: 0.1 mV = 1 mm = 1 small square.

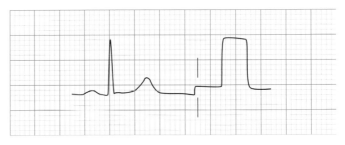

Figure 1.2 Standard calibration signal. Speed: 25 mm/s Gain: 10 mm/mV.

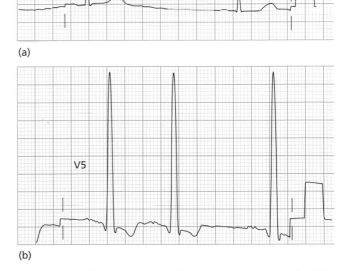

(a)

(b)

Figure 1.3 Role of body habitus and disease on the amplitude of the QRS complex. (a) Low amplitude complexes in an obese woman with hypothyroidism. (b) High amplitude complexes in a hypertensive man.

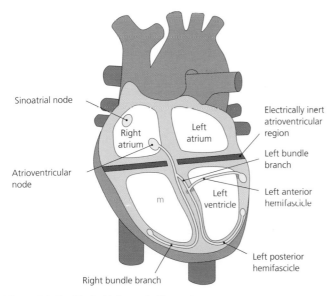

Figure 1.1 The His-Purkinje conduction system.

- Sinoatrial node
- Right atrium
- Left atrium
- Atrioventricular node
- Left ventricle
- Electrically inert atrioventricular region
- Left bundle branch
- Left anterior hemifascicle
- Left posterior hemifascicle
- Right bundle branch

Throughout this chapter the duration of waveforms will be expressed as 0.04 s = 1 mm = 1 small square

The amplitude of the waveform recorded in any lead may be influenced by the myocardial mass, the net vector of depolarisation, the thickness and properties of the intervening tissues, and the distance between the electrode and the myocardium. Patients with ventricular hypertrophy have a relatively large myocardial mass and are therefore likely to have high amplitude waveforms. In the presence of pericardial fluid, pulmonary emphysema, or obesity, there is increased resistance to current flow, and thus waveform amplitude is reduced.

The direction of the deflection on the electrocardiogram depends on whether the electrical impulse is travelling towards or away from a detecting electrode. By convention, an electrical impulse travelling directly towards the electrode produces an upright ("positive") deflection relative to the isoelectric baseline, whereas an impulse moving directly away from an electrode produces a downward ("negative") deflection relative to the baseline. When the wave of depolarisation is at right angles to the lead, an equiphasic deflection is produced.

The six chest leads (V1 to V6) "view" the heart in the horizontal plane. The information from the limb electrodes is combined to produce the six limb leads (I, II, III, aVR, aVL, and aVF), which view the heart in the vertical plane. The information from these 12 leads is combined to form a standard electrocardiogram.

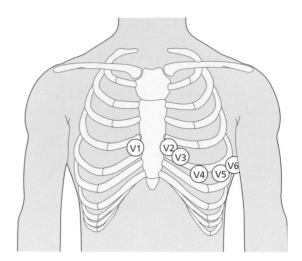

Figure 1.5 Position of the six chest electrodes for standard 12 lead electrocardiography. V1: right sternal edge, 4th intercostal space; V2: left sternal edge, 4th intercostal space; V3: between V2 and V4; V4: mid-clavicular line, 5th space; V5: anterior axillary line, horizontally in line with V4; V6: mid-axillary line, horizontally in line with V4.

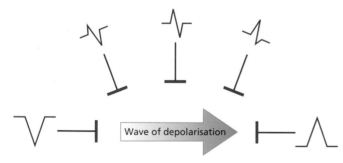

Figure 1.4 Wave of depolarisation. Shape of QRS complex in any lead depends on orientation of that lead to vector of depolarisation.

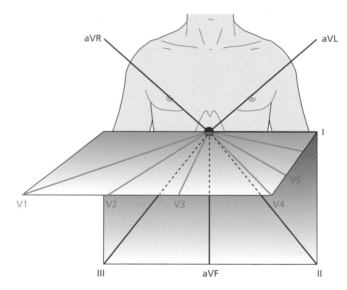

Figure 1.6 Vertical and horizontal perspective of the leads. The limb leads "view" the heart in the vertical plane and the chest leads in the horizontal plane.

The arrangement of the leads produces the following anatomical relationships: leads II, III, and aVF view the inferior surface of the heart; leads V1 to V4 view the anterior surface; leads I, aVL, V5, and V6 view the lateral surface; and leads V1 and aVR look through the right atrium directly into the cavity of the left ventricle.

Table 1.1 Anatomical relations of leads in a standard 12 lead electrocardiogram.

- II, III, and aVF: inferior surface of the heart
- V1 to V4: anterior surface
- I, aVL, V5, and V6: lateral surface
- V1 and aVR: right atrium and cavity of left ventricle

Waveforms mentioned in this chapter (for example, QRS complex, R wave, P wave) are explained in Chapter 2

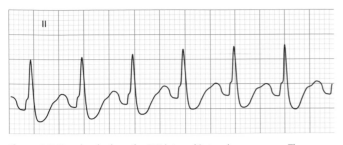

Figure 1.7 Regular rhythm: the R-R interval is two large squares. The rate is 150 beats/min (300/2=150).

Rate

The term tachycardia is used to describe a heart rate greater than 100 beats/min. A bradycardia is defined as a rate less than 60 beats/min (or <50 beats/min during sleep).

One large square of recording paper is equivalent to 0.2 seconds; there are five large squares per second and 300 per minute. Thus when the rhythm is regular and the paper speed is running at the standard rate of 25 mm/s, the heart rate can be calculated by counting the number of large squares between two consecutive R waves, and dividing this number into 300. Alternatively, the number of small squares between two consecutive R waves may be divided into 1500. Some countries use a paper speed of 50 mm/s as standard; the heart rate is calculated by dividing the number of large squares between R waves into 600, or the number of small squares into 3000.

"Rate rulers" are sometimes used to calculate heart rate; these are used to measure two or three consecutive R-R intervals, of which the average is expressed as the rate equivalent.

When using a rate ruler, take care to use the correct scale according to paper speed (25 or 50 mm/s); count the correct numbers of beats (for example, two or three); and restrict the technique to regular rhythms.

When an irregular rhythm is present, the heart rate may be calculated from the rhythm strip (see next section). It takes one second to record 2.5 cm of trace. The heart rate per minute can be calculated by counting the number of intervals between QRS complexes in 10 seconds (namely, 25 cm of recording paper) and multiplying by six.

Table 1.2 Cardinal features of sinus rhythm.

- The P wave is upright in leads I and II
- Each P wave is usually followed by a QRS complex
- The heart rate is 60-99 beats/min

Table 1.3 Normal findings in healthy individuals.

- Tall R waves
- Prominent U waves
- ST segment elevation (high take-off, benign early repolarisation)
- Exaggerated sinus arrhythmia
- Sinus bradycardia
- Wandering atrial pacemaker
- Wenckebach phenomenon
- Junctional rhythm
- 1st degree heart block

Rhythm

To assess the cardiac rhythm accurately, a prolonged recording from one lead is used to provide a rhythm strip. Lead II, which usually gives a good view of the P wave, is most commonly used to record the rhythm strip.

The term "sinus rhythm" is used when the rhythm originates in the sinus node and conducts to the ventricles.

Young, athletic people may display various other rhythms, particularly during sleep. Sinus arrhythmia is the variation in the heart rate that occurs during inspiration and expiration. There is "beat to beat" variation in the R R interval, the rate increasing with inspiration. It is a vagally mediated response to the increased volume of blood returning to the heart during inspiration.

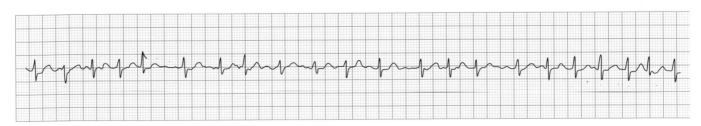

Figure 1.8 A standard rhythm strip is 25 cm long (that is, 10 seconds). The rate in this strip (showing an irregular rhythm with 21 intervals) is therefore 126 beats/min (6 × 21). Scale is slightly reduced here.

Cardiac axis

The cardiac axis refers to the mean direction of the wave of ventricular depolarisation in the vertical plane, measured from a zero reference point. The zero reference point looks at the heart from the same viewpoint as lead I. An axis lying above this line is given a negative number, and an axis lying below the line is given a positive number. Theoretically, the cardiac axis may lie anywhere between 180 and −180°. The normal range for the cardiac axis is between −30° and 90°. An axis lying beyond −30° is termed left axis deviation, whereas an axis >90° is termed right axis deviation.

Several methods can be used to calculate the cardiac axis, though occasionally it can prove extremely difficult to determine. The simplest method is by inspection of leads I, II, and III.

Table 1.4 Conditions for which determination of the axis is helpful in diagnosis.

- Conduction defects—for example, left anterior hemiblock
- Ventricular enlargement—for example, right ventricular hypertrophy
- Broad complex tachycardia—for example, bizarre axis suggestive of ventricular origin
- Congenital heart disease—for example, atrial septal defects
- Pre-excited conduction—for example, Wolff-Parkinson-White syndrome
- Pulmonary embolus

Table 1.5 Calculating the cardiac axis.

	Normal axis	Right axis deviation	Left axis deviation
Lead I	Positive	Negative	Positive
Lead II	Positive	Positive or negative	Negative
Lead III	Positive or negative	Positive	Negative

A more accurate estimate of the axis can be achieved if all six limb leads are examined. The hexaxial diagram shows each lead's view of the heart in the vertical plane. The direction of current flow is towards leads with a positive deflection, away from leads with a negative deflection, and at 90° to a lead with an equiphasic QRS complex. The axis is determined as follows:

- Choose the limb lead closest to being equiphasic. The axis lies about 90° to the right or left of this lead
- With reference to the hexaxial diagram, inspect the QRS complexes in the leads adjacent to the equiphasic lead. If the lead to the left side is positive, then the axis is 90° to the equiphasic lead towards the left. If the lead to the right side is positive, then the axis is 90° to the equiphasic lead towards the right.

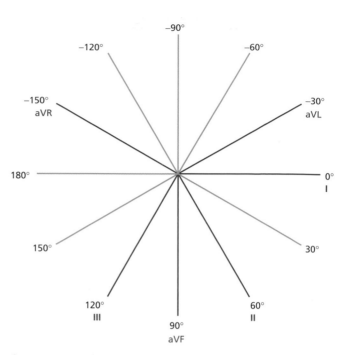

Figure 1.9 Hexaxial diagram (projection of six leads in vertical plane) showing each lead's view of the heart.

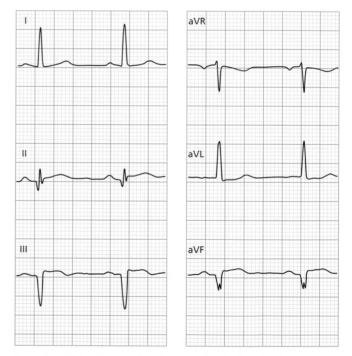

Figure 1.10 Determination of cardiac axis using the hexaxial diagram. Lead II (60°) is almost equiphasic and therefore the axis lies at 90° to this lead (that is 150° to the right or −30° to the left). Examination of the adjacent leads (leads I and III) shows that lead I is positive. The cardiac axis therefore lies at about −30°.

CHAPTER 2

Introduction. II—Basic Terminology

Steve Meek, Francis Morris

This chapter explains the genesis of and normal values for the individual components of the wave forms that are seen in an electrocardiogram. To recognise electrocardiographic abnormalities the range of normal wave patterns must be understood.

P wave

The sinoatrial node lies high in the wall of the right atrium and initiates atrial depolarisation, producing the P wave on the electrocardiogram. Although the atria are anatomically two distinct chambers, electrically they act almost as one. They have relatively little muscle and generate a single, small P wave. P wave amplitude rarely exceeds two and a half small squares (0.25 mV). The duration of the P wave should not exceed three small squares (0.12 s).

The wave of depolarisation is directed inferiorly and towards the left, and thus the P wave tends to be upright in leads I and II and inverted in lead aVR. Sinus P waves are usually most prominently seen in leads II and V1. A negative P wave in lead I may be due to incorrect recording of the electrocardiogram (that is, with transposition of the left and right arm electrodes), dextrocardia, or abnormal atrial rhythms.

The P wave in V1 is often biphasic. Early right atrial forces are directed anteriorly, giving rise to an initial positive deflection; these are followed by left atrial forces travelling posteriorly, producing a later negative deflection. A large negative deflection (area of more than one small square) suggests left atrial enlargement.

Normal P waves may have a slight notch, particularly in the precordial (chest) leads. Bifid P waves result from slight asynchrony

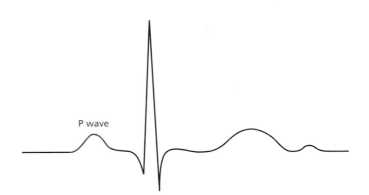

P wave

Figure 2.2 Complex showing P wave highlighted.

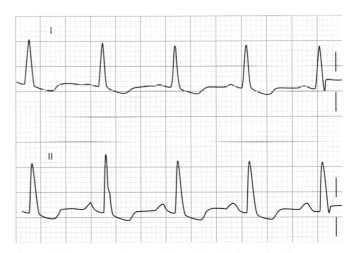

I

II

Figure 2.3 P waves usually more obvious in lead II than in lead I.

Table 2.1 Characteristics of the P wave.

- Positive in leads I and II
- Best seen in leads II and V1
- Commonly biphasic in lead V1
- < 3 small squares in duration
- < 2.5 small squares in amplitude

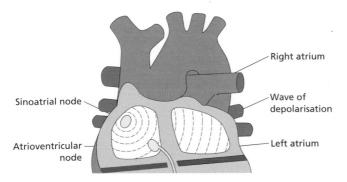

Right atrium

Sinoatrial node

Wave of depolarisation

Atrioventricular node

Left atrium

Figure 2.1 Atrial depolarisation gives rise to the P wave.

between right and left atrial depolarisation. A pronounced notch with a peak-to-peak interval of >1 mm (0.04 s) is usually pathological, and is seen in association with a left atrial abnormality—for example, in mitral stenosis.

PR interval

After the P wave there is a brief return to the isoelectric line, resulting in the "PR segment." During this time the electrical impulse is conducted through the atrioventricular node, the bundle of His and bundle branches, and the Purkinje fibres.

The PR interval is the time between the onset of atrial depolarisation and the onset of ventricular depolarisation, and it is measured from the beginning of the P wave to the first deflection of the QRS complex (see next section), whether this be a Q wave or an R wave. The normal duration of the PR interval is three to five small squares (0.12-0.20 s). Abnormalities of the conducting system may lead to transmission delays, prolonging the PR interval.

QRS complex

The QRS complex represents the electrical forces generated by ventricular depolarisation. With normal intraventricular conduction, depolarisation occurs in an efficient, rapid fashion. The duration of the QRS complex is measured in the lead with the widest complex and should not exceed two and a half small squares (0.10 s). Delays in ventricular depolarisation—for example, bundle branch block—give rise to abnormally wide QRS complexes (≥0.12 s).

The depolarisation wave travels through the interventricular septum via the bundle of His and bundle branches and reaches the ventricular myocardium via the Purkinje fibre network. The left side of the septum depolarises first, and the impulse then spreads towards the right. Lead V1 lies immediately to the right of the septum and thus registers an initial small positive deflection (R wave) as the depolarisation wave travels towards this lead.

When the wave of septal depolarisation travels away from the recording electrode, the first deflection inscribed is negative. Thus small "septal" Q waves are often present in the lateral leads, usually leads I, aVL, V5, and V6.

These non-pathological Q waves are less than two small squares deep and less than one small square wide, and should be < 25% of the amplitude of the corresponding R wave.

The wave of depolarisation reaches the endocardium at the apex of the ventricles, and then travels to the epicardium, spreading outwards in all directions. Depolarisation of the right and left ventricles produces opposing electrical vectors, but the left ventricle has the larger muscle mass and its depolarisation dominates the electrocardiogram.

In the precordial leads, QRS morphology changes depending on whether the depolarisation forces are moving towards or away from a lead. The forces generated by the free wall of the left ventricle predominate, and therefore in lead V1 a small R wave is followed by a large negative deflection (S wave). The R wave in the precordial leads steadily increases in amplitude from lead V1 to V6, with a corresponding decrease in S wave depth, culminating in a predominantly positive complex in V6. Thus, the QRS complex

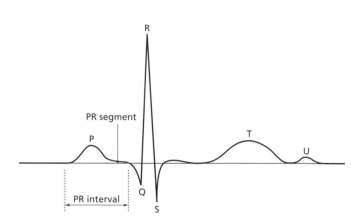

Figure 2.4 Normal duration of PR interval is 0.12-0.20 s (three to five small squares).

Table 2.2 Nomenclature in QRS complexes.

Q wave: Any initial negative deflection
R wave: Any positive deflection
S wave: Any negative deflection after an R wave

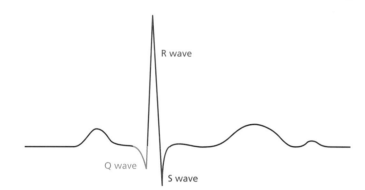

Figure 2.5 Composition of QRS complex.

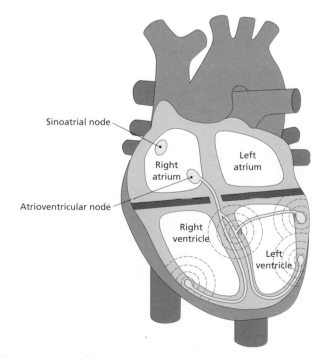

Figure 2.6 Wave of depolarisation spreading throughout ventricles gives rise to QRS complex.

gradually changes from being predominantly negative in lead V1 to being predominantly positive in lead V6. The lead with an equiphasic QRS complex is located over the transition zone; this lies between leads V3 and V4, but shifts towards the left with age.

The height of the R wave is variable and increases progressively across the precordial leads; it is usually < 27 mm in leads V5 and V6. The R wave in lead V6, however, is often smaller than the R wave in V5, since the V6 electrode is further from the left ventricle.

The S wave is deepest in the right precordial leads; it decreases in amplitude across the precordium, and is often absent in leads V5 and V6. The depth of the S wave should not exceed 30 mm in a normal individual, although S waves and R waves > 30 mm are occasionally recorded in normal young male adults.

ST segment

The QRS complex terminates at the J point or ST junction. The ST segment lies between the J point and the beginning of the T wave, and represents the period between the end of ventricular depolarisation and the beginning of repolarisation.

The ST segment should be level with the subsequent "TP segment" and is normally fairly flat, though it may slope upwards slightly before merging with the T wave.

In leads V1 to V3 the rapidly ascending S wave merges directly with the T wave, making the J point indistinct and the ST segment difficult to identify. This produces elevation of the ST segment, and this is known as "high take-off."

Non-pathological elevation of the ST segment is also associated with benign early repolarisation (see Chapters 8 and 9 on acute myocardial infarction), which is particularly common in young men, athletes, and black people.

Interpretation of subtle abnormalities of the ST segment is one of the more difficult areas of clinical electrocardiography; nevertheless, any elevation or depression of the ST segment must be explained rather than dismissed.

T wave

Ventricular repolarisation produces the T wave. The normal T wave is asymmetrical, the first half having a more gradual slope than the second half.

T wave orientation usually corresponds with that of the QRS complex, and thus is inverted in lead aVR, and may be inverted in lead III. T wave inversion in lead V1 is also common. It is occasionally accompanied by T wave inversion in lead V2, though isolated

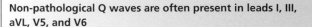

Non-pathological Q waves are often present in leads I, III, aVL, V5, and V6

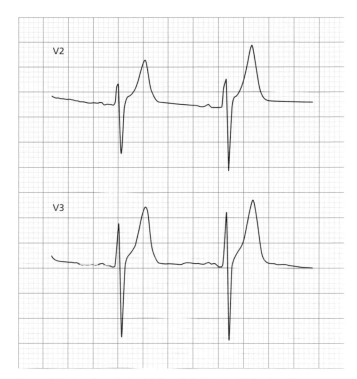

Figure 2.8 Complexes in leads V2 and V3 showing high take-off.

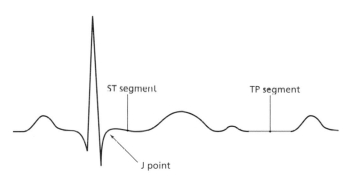

Figure 2.9 The ST segment should be in the same horizontal plane as the TP segment; the J point is the point of inflection between the S wave and ST segment.

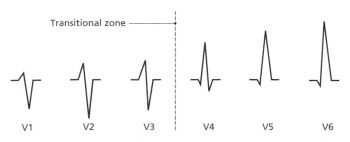

Figure 2.7 Typical change in morphology of QRS complex from leads V1 to V6.

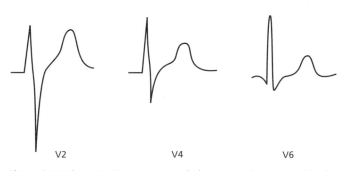

Figure 2.10 Change in ST segment morphology across the precordial leads.

> **The T wave should generally be at least 1/8 but less than 2/3 of the amplitude of the corresponding R wave; T wave amplitude rarely exceeds 10 mm**

T wave inversion in lead V2 is abnormal. T wave inversion in two or more of the right precordial leads is known as a persistent juvenile pattern; it is more common in black people. The presence of symmetrical, inverted T waves is highly suggestive of myocardial ischaemia, though asymmetrical inverted T waves are frequently a non-specific finding.

No widely accepted criteria exist regarding T wave amplitude. As a general rule, T wave amplitude corresponds with the amplitude of the preceding R wave, though the tallest T waves are seen in leads V3 and V4. Tall T waves may be seen in acute myocardial ischaemia and are a feature of hyperkalaemia.

QT interval

The QT interval is measured from the beginning of the QRS complex to the end of the T wave and represents the total time taken for depolarisation and repolarisation of the ventricles.

The QT interval lengthens as the heart rate slows, and thus when measuring the QT interval the rate must be taken into account. As a general guide the QT interval should be 0.35–0.45 s, and should not be more than half of the interval between adjacent R waves (R-R interval). The QT interval increases slightly with age and tends to be longer in women than in men. Bazett's correction is used to calculate the QT interval corrected for heart rate (QTc): $QTc = QT/\sqrt{R\text{-}R}$ (seconds).

Prominent U waves can easily be mistaken for T waves, leading to overestimation of the QT interval. This mistake can be avoided by identifying a lead where U waves are not prominent—for example, lead aVL.

U wave

The U wave is a small deflection that follows the T wave. It is generally upright except in the aVR lead and is often most prominent in leads V2 to V4. U waves result from repolarisation of the mid-myocardial cells—that is, those between the endocardium and the epicardium—and the His-Purkinje system.

Many electrocardiograms have no discernible U waves. Prominent U waves may be found in athletes and are associated with hypokalaemia and hypercalcaemia.

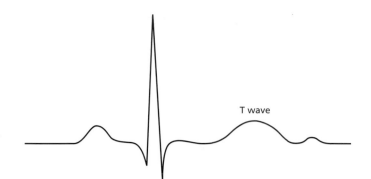

Figure 2.11 Complex showing T wave highlighted.

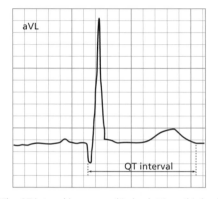

Figure 2.12 The QT interval is measured in lead aVL as this lead does not have prominent U waves (diagram is scaled up).

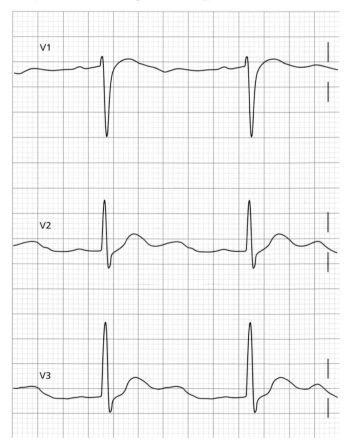

Figure 2.13 Obvious U waves in leads V1 to V3 in patient with hypokalaemia.

CHAPTER 3

Bradycardias and Atrioventricular Conduction Block

David Da Costa, William J Brady, June Edhouse

By arbitrary definition, a bradycardia is a heart rate of < 60 beats/min. A bradycardia may be a normal physiological phenomenon or result from a cardiac or non-cardiac disorder.

Sinus bradycardia

Sinus bradycardia is common in normal individuals during sleep and in those with high vagal tone, such as athletes and young healthy adults. The electrocardiogram shows a P wave before every QRS complex, with a normal P wave axis (that is, upright P wave in lead II). The PR interval is at least 0.12 s.

The commonest pathological cause of sinus bradycardia is acute myocardial infarction. Sinus bradycardia is particularly associated with inferior myocardial infarction as the inferior myocardial wall and the sinoatrial and atrioventricular nodes are usually all supplied by the right coronary artery.

Sick sinus syndrome

Sick sinus syndrome is the result of dysfunction of the sinoatrial node, with impairment of its ability to generate and conduct impulses. It usually results from idiopathic fibrosis of the node but is also associated with myocardial ischaemia, digoxin, and cardiac surgery.

The possible electrocardiographic features include persistent sinus bradycardia, periods of sinoatrial block, sinus arrest, junctional or ventricular escape rhythms, tachycardia-bradycardia syndrome, paroxysmal atrial flutter, and atrial fibrillation. The commonest electrocardiographic feature is an inappropriate, persistent, and often severe sinus bradycardia.

> Many patients tolerate heart rates of 40 beats/min surprisingly well, but at lower rates symptoms are likely to include dizziness, near syncope, syncope, ischaemic chest pain, Stokes-Adams attacks, and hypoxic seizures

Table 3.1 Pathological causes of sinus bradycardia.

- Acute myocardial infarction
- Drugs—for example, β blockers, digoxin, amiodarone
- Obstructive jaundice
- Raised intracranial pressure
- Sick sinus syndrome
- Hypothermia
- Hypothyroidism

Table 3.2 Conditions associated with sinoatrial node dysfunction.

- Age
- Idiopathic fibrosis
- Ischaemia, including myocardial infarction
- High vagal tone
- Myocarditis
- Digoxin toxicity

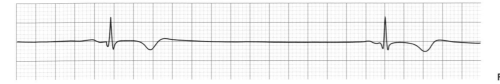

Figure 3.1 Severe sinus bradycardia.

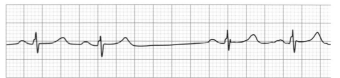

Figure 3.2 Sinoatrial block (note the pause is twice the P-P interval).

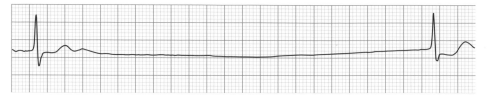

Figure 3.3 Sinus arrest with pause of 4.4 s before generation and conduction of a junctional escape beat.

Sinoatrial block is characterised by a transient failure of impulse conduction to the atrial myocardium, resulting in intermittent pauses between P waves. The pauses are the length of two or more P-P intervals.

Sinus arrest occurs when there is transient cessation of impulse formation at the sinoatrial node; it manifests as a prolonged pause without P wave activity. The pause is unrelated to the length of the P-P cycle.

Escape rhythms are the result of spontaneous activity from a subsidiary pacemaker, located in the atria, atrioventricular junction, or ventricles. They take over when normal impulse formation or conduction fails and may be associated with any profound bradycardia.

Atrioventricular conduction block

Atrioventricular conduction can be delayed, intermittently blocked, or completely blocked—classified correspondingly as first, second, or third degree block.

First degree block

In first degree block there is a delay in conduction of the atrial impulse to the ventricles, usually at the level of the atrioventricular node. This results in prolongation of the PR interval to >0.2 s. A QRS complex follows each P wave, and the PR interval remains constant.

Second degree block

In second degree block there is intermittent failure of conduction between the atria and ventricles. Some P waves are not followed by a QRS complex.

There are three types of second degree block. Mobitz type I block (Wenckebach phenomenon) is usually at the level of the atrioventricular node, producing intermittent failure of transmission of the atrial impulse to the ventricles. The initial PR interval is normal but progressively lengthens with each successive beat until eventually atrioventricular transmission is blocked completely and the P wave is not followed by a QRS complex. The PR interval then returns to normal, and the cycle repeats.

Mobitz type II block is less common but is more likely to produce symptoms. There is intermittent failure of conduction of P waves. The PR interval is constant, though it may be normal or prolonged. The block is often at the level of the bundle branches and is therefore associated with wide QRS complexes. 2:1 atrioventricular block is difficult to classify, but it is usually a Wenckebach variant. High degree atrioventricular block, which occurs when a QRS complex is seen only after every three, four, or more P waves, may progress to complete third degree atrioventricular block.

> **A junctional escape beat has a normal QRS complex shape with a rate of 40-60 beats/min. A ventricular escape rhythm has broad complexes and is slow (15-40 beats/min)**

Table 3.3 Tachycardia-bradycardia syndrome.

- Common in sick sinus syndrome
- Characterised by bursts of atrial tachycardia interspersed with periods of bradycardia
- Paroxysmal atrial flutter or fibrillation may also occur, and
- cardioversion may be followed by a severe bradycardia

Table 3.4 Causes of atrioventricular conduction block.

- Myocardial ischaemia or infarction
- Degeneration of the His-Purkinje system
- Infection—for example, Lyme disease, diphtheria
- Immunological disorders—for example, systemic lupus erythematosus
- Surgery
- Congenital disorders

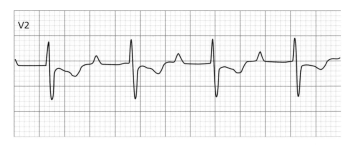

Figure 3.4 First degree heart (atrioventricular) block.

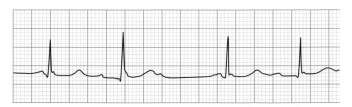

Figure 3.5 Mobitz type I block (Wenckebach phenomenon).

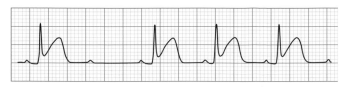

Figure 3.6 Mobitz type II block—a complication of an inferior myocardial infarction. The PR interval is identical before and after the P wave that is not conducted.

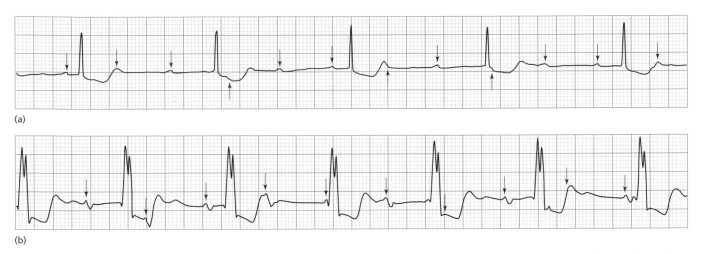

(a)

(b)

Figure 3.7 Third degree heart block. A pacemaker in the bundle of His produces a narrow QRS complex (a), whereas more distal pacemakers tend to produce broader complexes (b). Arrows show P waves.

Third degree block

In third degree block there is complete failure of conduction between the atria and ventricles, with complete independence of atrial and ventricular contractions. The P waves bear no relation to the QRS complexes and usually proceed at a faster rate.

A subsidiary pacemaker triggers ventricular contractions, though occasionally no escape rhythm occurs and asystolic arrest ensues. The rate and QRS morphology of the escape rhythm vary depending on the site of the pacemaker.

Bundle branch block and fascicular block

The bundle of His divides into the right and left bundle branches. The left bundle branch then splits into anterior and posterior hemifascicles. Conduction blocks in any of these structures produce characteristic electrocardiographic changes.

Right bundle branch block

In most cases right bundle branch block has a pathological cause though it is also seen in healthy individuals.

Table 3.5 Diagnostic criteria for right bundle branch block.

- QRS duration ≥0.12 s
- A secondary R wave (R') in V1 or V2
- Wide slurred S wave in leads I, V5, and V6

Associated feature
- ST segment depression and T wave inversion in the right precordial leads

When conduction in the right bundle branch is blocked, depolarisation of the right ventricle is delayed. The left ventricle depolarises in the normal way and thus the early part of the QRS complex appears normal. The wave of depolarisation then spreads to the right ventricle through non-specialised conducting tissue, with slow depolarisation of the right ventricle in a left to right direction. As left ventricular depolarisation is complete, the forces of right ventricular depolarisation are unopposed. Thus the later part

Table 3.6 Conditions associated with right bundle branch block.

- Rheumatic heart disease
- Cor pulmonale/right ventricular hypertrophy
- Myocarditis or cardiomyopathy
- Ischaemic heart disease
- Degenerative disease of the conduction system
- Pulmonary embolus
- Congenital heart disease—for example, in atrial septal defects

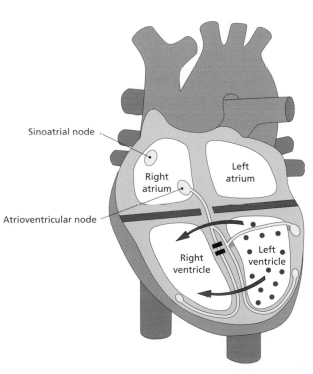

Figure 3.8 Right bundle branch block, showing the wave of depolarisation spreading to the right ventricle through non-specialised conducting tissue.

of the QRS complex is abnormal; the right precordial leads have a prominent and late R wave, and the left precordial and limb leads have a terminal S wave. These terminal deflections are wide and slurred. Abnormal ventricular depolarisation is associated with secondary repolarisation changes, giving rise to changes in the ST-T waves in the right chest leads.

Left bundle branch block

Left bundle branch block is most commonly caused by coronary artery disease, hypertensive heart disease, or dilated cardiomyopathy. It is unusual for left bundle branch block to exist in the absence of organic disease.

The left bundle branch is supplied by both the anterior descending artery (a branch of the left coronary artery) and the right coronary artery. Thus patients who develop left bundle branch block generally have extensive disease. This type of block is seen in 2-4% of patients with acute myocardial infarction and is usually associated with anterior infarction.

Table 3.7 Diagnostic criteria for left bundle branch block.

- QRS duration of ≥0.12 s
- Broad monophasic R wave in leads 1, V5, and V6
- Absence of Q waves in leads V5 and V6

Associated features
- Displacement of ST segment and T wave in an opposite direction to the dominant deflection of the QRS complex (appropriate discordance)
- Poor R wave progression in the chest leads
- RS complex, rather than monophasic complex, in leads V5 and V6
- Left axis deviation—common but not invariable finding

In the normal heart, septal depolarisation proceeds from left to right, producing Q waves in the left chest leads (septal Q waves). In left bundle branch block the direction of depolarisation of the intraventricular septum is reversed; the septal Q waves are lost and replaced with R waves. The delay in left ventricular depolarisation increases the duration of the QRS complex to >0.12 s. Abnormal ventricular depolarisation leads to secondary repolarisation changes. ST segment depression and T wave inversion are seen in leads with a dominant R wave. ST segment elevation and positive T waves are seen in leads with a dominant S wave. Thus there is discordance between the QRS complex and the ST segment and T wave.

Fascicular blocks

Block of the left anterior and posterior hemifascicles gives rise to the hemiblocks. Left anterior hemiblock is characterised by a mean frontal plane axis more leftward than −30° (abnormal left axis deviation) in the absence of an inferior myocardial infarction or other cause of left axis deviation. Left posterior hemiblock is characterised by a mean frontal plane axis of >90° in the absence of other causes of right axis deviation.

Bifascicular block is the combination of right bundle branch block and left anterior or posterior hemiblock. The electrocardiogram shows right bundle branch block with left or right axis deviation. Right bundle branch block with left anterior hemiblock is the commonest type of bifascicular block. The left posterior fascicle is

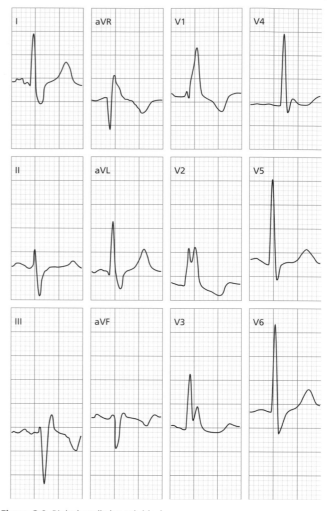

Figure 3.9 Right bundle branch block.

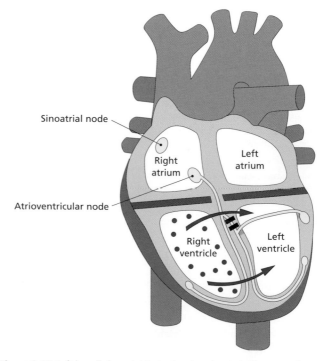

Figure 3.10 Left bundle branch block, showing depolarisation spreading from the right to left ventricle.

fairly stout and more resistant to damage, so right bundle branch block with left posterior hemiblock is rarely seen.

Trifascicular block is present when bifascicular block is associated with first degree heart block. If conduction in the dysfunctional fascicle also fails completely, complete heart block ensues.

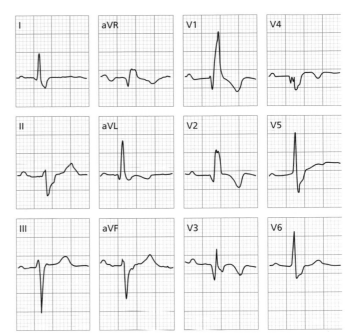

Figure 3.12 Trifascicular block (right bundle branch block, left anterior hemiblock, and first degree heart block).

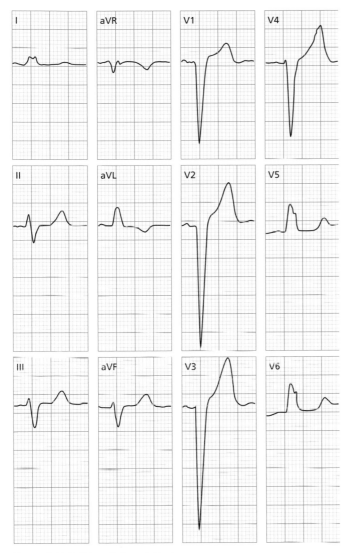

Figure 3.11 Left bundle branch block.

CHAPTER 4

Atrial Arrhythmias

Steve Goodacre, Richard Irons

In adults a tachycardia is any heart rate greater than 100 beats per minute. Supraventricular tachycardias may be divided into two distinct groups depending on whether they arise from the atria or the atrioventricular junction. This chapter will consider those arising from the atria: sinus tachycardia, atrial fibrillation, atrial flutter, and atrial tachycardia. Tachycardias arising from re-entry circuits in the atrioventricular junction will be considered in the next chapter.

Clinical relevance

The clinical importance of a tachycardia in an individual patient is related to the ventricular rate, the presence of any underlying heart disease, and the integrity of cardiovascular reflexes. Coronary blood flow occurs during diastole, and as the heart rate increases diastole shortens. In the presence of coronary atherosclerosis, blood flow may become critical and anginal-type chest pain may result. Similar chest pain, which is not related to myocardial ischaemia, may also occur. Reduced cardiac performance produces symptoms of faintness or syncope and leads to increased sympathetic stimulation, which may increase the heart rate further.

As a general rule the faster the ventricular rate, the more likely the presence of symptoms—for example, chest pain, faintness, and breathlessness. Urgent treatment is needed for severely symptomatic patients with a narrow complex tachycardia.

Electrocardiographic features

Differentiation between different types of supraventricular tachycardia may be difficult, particularly when ventricular rates exceed 150 beats/min.

Knowledge of the electrophysiology of these arrhythmias will assist correct identification. Evaluation of atrial activity on the electrocardiogram is crucial in this process. Analysis of the ventricular rate and rhythm may also be helpful, although this rate will depend on the degree of atrioventricular block.

Increasing atrioventricular block by manoeuvres such as carotid sinus massage or administration of intravenous adenosine may be of diagnostic value as slowing the ventricular rate allows more accurate visualisation of atrial activity. Such manoeuvres will not usually stop the tachycardia, however, unless it is due to re-entry involving the atrioventricular node.

Sinus tachycardia

Sinus tachycardia is usually a physiological response but may be precipitated by sympathomimetic drugs or endocrine disturbances.

The rate rarely exceeds 200 beats/min in adults. The rate increases gradually and may show beat to beat variation. Each P wave is followed by a QRS complex. P wave morphology and axis are normal, although the height of the P wave may increase with the heart rate and the PR interval will shorten. With a fast tachycardia the P wave may become lost in the preceding T wave.

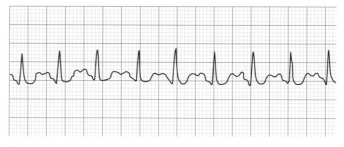

Figure 4.1 Sinus tachycardia.

Table 4.1 Supraventricular tachycardias.

From the atria or sinoatrial node
- Sinus tachycardia
- Atrial fibrillation
- Atrial flutter
- Atrial tachycardia

From the atrioventricular node
- Atrioventricular re-entrant tachycardia
- Atrioventricular nodal re-entrant tachycardia

Electrocardiographic analysis should include measurement of the ventricular rate, assessment of the ventricular rhythm, identification of P, F, or f waves , measurement of the atrial rate, and establishment of the relation of P waves to the ventricular complexes

Recognition of the underlying cause usually makes diagnosis of sinus tachycardia easy. A persistent tachycardia in the absence of an obvious underlying cause should prompt consideration of atrial flutter or atrial tachycardia.

Rarely the sinus tachycardia may be due to a re-entry phenomenon in the sinoatrial node. This is recognised by abrupt onset and termination, a very regular rate, and absence of an underlying physiological stimulus. The electrocardiographic characteristics are otherwise identical. The rate is usually 130-140 beats/min, and vagal manoeuvres may be successful in stopping the arrhythmia.

Atrial fibrillation

This is the most common sustained arrhythmia. Overall prevalence is 1% to 1.5%, but prevalence increases with age, affecting about 10% of people aged over 70. Causes are varied, although many cases are idiopathic. Prognosis is related to the underlying cause; it is excellent when due to idiopathic atrial fibrillation and relatively poor when due to ischaemic cardiomyopathy.

Atrial fibrillation is caused by multiple re-entrant circuits or "wavelets" of activation sweeping around the atrial myocardium. These are often triggered by rapid firing foci. Atrial fibrillation is seen on the electrocardiogram as a wavy, irregular baseline made up of f (fibrillation) waves discharging at a frequency of 350 to 600 beats/min. The amplitude of these waves varies between leads but may be so coarse that they are mistaken for flutter waves.

Conduction of atrial impulses to the ventricles is variable and unpredictable. Only a few of the impulses transmit through the atrioventricular node to produce an irregular ventricular response. This combination of absent P waves, fine baseline f wave oscillations, and irregular ventricular complexes is characteristic of atrial fibrillation. The ventricular rate depends on the degree of atrioventricular conduction, and with normal conduction it varies between 100 and 180 beats/min. Slower rates suggest a higher

Table 4.2 Electrocardiographic characteristics of atrial arrhythmias.

Sinus tachycardia
- P waves have normal morphology
- Atrial rate 100-200 beats/min
- Regular ventricular rhythm
- Ventricular rate 100-200 beats/min
- One P wave precedes every QRS complex

Atrial tachycardia
- Abnormal P wave morphology
- Atrial rate 100-250 beats/min
- Ventricular rhythm usually regular
- Variable ventricular rate

Atrial flutter
- Undulating saw-toothed baseline F (flutter) waves
- Atrial rate 250-350 beats/min
- Regular ventricular rhythm
- Ventricular rate typically 150 beats/min (with 2:1 atrioventricular block)
- 4:1 is also common (3:1 and 1:1 block uncommon)

Atrial fibrillation
- P waves absent; oscillating baseline f (fibrillation) waves
- Atrial rate 350-600 beats/min
- Irregular ventricular rhythm
- Ventricular rate 100-180 beats/min

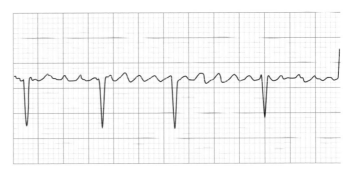

Figure 4.3 Atrial fibrillation waves seen in lead V1.

Table 4.3 Causes of sinus tachycardia.

Physiological—Exertion, anxiety, pain
Pathological—Fever, anaemia, hypovolaemia, hypoxia
Endocrine—Thyrotoxicosis
Pharmacological—Adrenaline as a result of phaeochromocytoma; salbutamol; alcohol, caffeine

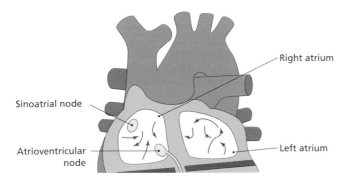

Figure 4.2 Atrial fibrillation is the result of multiple wavelets of depolarisation (shown by arrows) moving around the atria chaotically, rarely completing a re-entrant circuit.

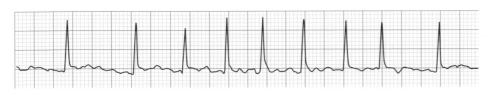

Figure 4.4 Rhythm strip in atrial fibrillation.

degree of atrioventricular block or the patient may be taking medication such as digoxin.

Fast atrial fibrillation may be difficult to distinguish from other tachycardias. The R-R interval remains irregular, however, and the overall rate often fluctuates. Mapping R waves against a piece of paper or with calipers usually confirms the diagnosis.

Atrial fibrillation may be paroxysmal, persistent, or permanent. It may be precipitated by an atrial extrasystole or result from degeneration of other supraventricular tachycardias, particularly atrial tachycardia and/or flutter.

Atrial flutter

Atrial flutter is due to a re-entry circuit in the right atrium with secondary activation of the left atrium. This produces atrial contractions at a rate of about 300 beats/min—seen on the electrocardiogram as flutter (F) waves. These are broad and appear saw-toothed and are best seen in the inferior leads and in lead V1.

The ventricular rate depends on conduction through the atrioventricular node. Typically 2:1 block (atrial rate to ventricular rate) occurs, giving a ventricular rate of 150 beats/min. Identification of

a regular tachycardia with this rate should prompt the diagnosis of atrial flutter. The non-conducting flutter waves are often mistaken for or merged with T waves and become apparent only if the block is increased. Manoeuvres that induce transient atrioventricular block may allow identification of flutter waves.

Table 4.4 Causes of atrial fibrillation.

- Ischaemic heart disease
- Hypertensive heart disease
- Rheumatic heart disease
- Thyrotoxicosis
- Alcohol misuse (acute or chronic)
- Cardiomyopathy (dilated or hypertrophic)
- Sick sinus syndrome
- Post-cardiac surgery
- Chronic pulmonary disease
- Idiopathic (lone)

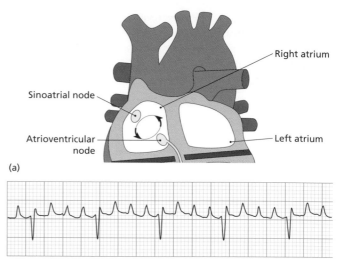

(a)

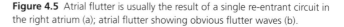

(b)

Figure 4.5 Atrial flutter is usually the result of a single re-entrant circuit in the right atrium (a); atrial flutter showing obvious flutter waves (b).

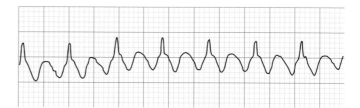

Figure 4.6 Rhythm strip in atrial flutter (rate 150 beats/min).

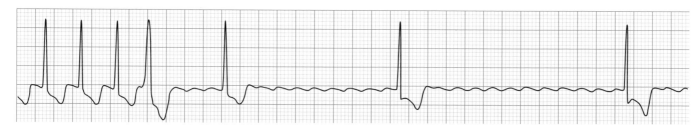

Figure 4.7 Atrial flutter (rate 150 beats/min) with increasing block (flutter waves revealed after administration of adenosine).

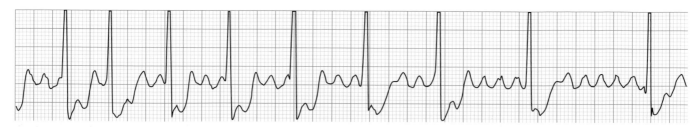

Figure 4.8 Atrial flutter with variable block.

The causes of atrial flutter are similar to those of atrial fibrillation, although idiopathic atrial flutter is uncommon. It may convert into atrial fibrillation over time or, after administration of drugs such as digoxin.

Atrial tachycardia

Atrial tachycardia typically arises from an ectopic source in the atrial muscle and produces an atrial rate of 150-250 beats/min—slower than that of atrial flutter. The P waves may be abnormally shaped depending on the site of the ectopic pacemaker.

The ventricular rate depends on the degree of atrioventricular block, but when 1:1 conduction occurs a rapid ventricular response

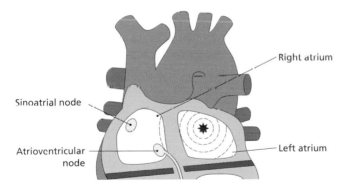

Figure 4.9 Atrial tachycardia with 2:1 block (note the inverted P waves).

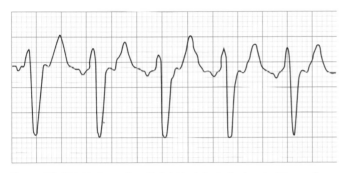

Figrue 4.10 Atrial tachycardia is initiated by an ectopic atrial focus (the P wave morphology therefore differs from that of sinus rhythm).

Table 4.5 Types of atrial tachycardia.

- Benign
- Incessant ectopic
- Multifocal
- Atrial tachycardia with block (digoxin toxicity)

may result. Increasing the degree of block with carotid sinus massage or adenosine may aid the diagnosis.

There are four commonly recognised types of atrial tachycardia. Benign atrial tachycardia is a common arrhythmia in elderly people. It is paroxysmal in nature, has an atrial rate of 80-140 beats/min and an abrupt onset and cessation, and is brief in duration.

Incessant ectopic atrial tachycardia is a rare chronic arrhythmia in children and young adults. The rate depends on the underlying sympathetic tone and is characteristically 100-160 beats/min. It can be difficult to distinguish from a sinus tachycardia. Diagnosis is important as it may lead to dilated cardiomyopathy if left untreated.

Multifocal atrial tachycardia occurs when multiple sites in the atria are discharging and is due to increased automaticity. It is characterised by P waves of varying morphologies and PR intervals of different lengths on the electrocardiographic trace. The ventricular rate is irregular. It can be distinguished from atrial fibrillation by an isoelectric baseline between the P waves. It is typically seen in association with chronic pulmonary disease. Other causes include hypoxia or digoxin toxicity.

Atrial tachycardia with atrioventricular block is typically seen with digoxin toxicity. The ventricular rhythm is usually regular but may be irregular if atrioventricular block is variable. Although often referred to as "paroxysmal atrial tachycardia with block" this arrhythmia is usually sustained.

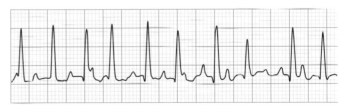

Figure 4.11 Multifocal atrial tachycardia.

Table 4.6 Conditions associated with atrial tachycardia.

- Cardiomyopathy
- Chronic obstructive pulmonary disease
- Ischaemic heart disease
- Rheumatic heart disease
- Sick sinus syndrome
- Digoxin toxicity

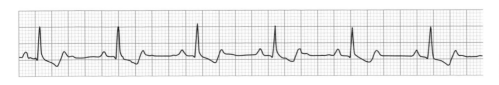

Figure 4.12 Atrial tachycardia with 2:1 block in patient with digoxin toxicity.

CHAPTER 5
Junctional Tachycardias

Demas Esberger, Sallyann Jones, Francis Morris

Any tachyarrhythmia arising from the atria or the atrioventricular junction is a supraventricular tachycardia. In clinical practice, however, the term supraventricular tachycardia is reserved for atrial tachycardias and arrhythmias arising from the region of the atrioventricular junction as a result of a re-entry mechanism (junctional tachycardias). The most common junctional tachycardias are atrioventricular nodal re-entrant tachycardia and atrioventricular re-entrant tachycardia.

Atrioventricular nodal re-entrant tachycardia

This is the most common cause of paroxysmal regular narrow complex tachycardia. Affected individuals are usually young and healthy with no organic heart disease.

Mechanism

In atrioventricular nodal re-entrant tachycardia there are two functionally and anatomically different distinct pathways in the atrioventricular node, with different conduction velocities and different refractory periods. They share a final common pathway through the lower part of the atrioventricular node and bundle of His. One pathway is relatively fast and has a long refractory period; the other pathway is slow with a short refractory period. In sinus rhythm the atrial impulse is conducted through the fast pathway and depolarises the ventricles. The impulse also travels down the slow pathway but terminates because the final common pathway is refractory.

The slow pathway has a short refractory period and recovers first. An atrioventricular nodal re-entrant tachycardia is initiated, for example, if a premature atrial beat occurs at the critical moment when the fast pathway is still refractory. The impulse is conducted through the slow pathway and is then propagated in a retrograde fashion up the fast pathway, which has by now recovered from its refractory period. Thus a re-entry through the circuit is created.

This type of "slow-fast" re-entry circuit is found in 90% of patients with atrioventricular nodal re-entrant tachycardia. Most of the rest have a fast-slow circuit, in which the re-entrant

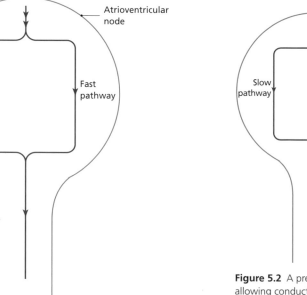

Figure 5.1 Mechanism of atrioventricular nodal re-entrant tachycardia showing the slow and fast conduction routes and the final common pathway through the lower part of the atrioventricular node and bundle of His.

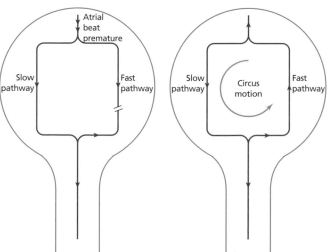

Figure 5.2 A premature atrial impulse finds the fast pathway refractory, allowing conduction only down the slow pathway (left). By the time the impulse reaches the His bundle, the fast pathway may have recovered, allowing retrograde conduction back up to the atria—the resultant "circus movement" gives rise to slow-fast atrioventricular nodal re-entrant tachycardia (right).

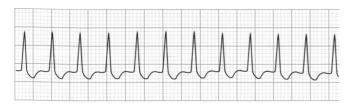

Figure 5.3 An atrioventricular nodal re-entrant tachycardia.

tachycardia is initiated by a premature ventricular contraction, and the impulse travels retrogradely up the slow pathway. This uncommon form of atrioventricular nodal re-entrant tachycardia is often sustained for very long periods and is then known as permanent junctional re-entrant tachycardia and is recognised by a long RP[1] interval.

Electrocardiographic findings

During sinus rhythm the electrocardiogram is normal. During the tachycardia the rhythm is regular, with narrow QRS complexes and a rate of 130-250 beats/min. Atrial conduction proceeds in a retrograde fashion producing inverted P waves in leads II, III, and aVF. However, since atrial and ventricular depolarisation often occurs simultaneously, the P waves are frequently buried in the QRS complex and may be totally obscured. A P wave may be seen distorting the last part of the QRS complex giving rise to a "pseudo" S wave in the inferior leads and a "pseudo" R wave in V1.

> **Fast-slow atrioventricular nodal re-entrant tachycardia is known as long RP[1] tachycardia, and it may be difficult to distinguish from an atrial tachycardia**

In the relatively uncommon fast-slow atrioventricular nodal re-entrant tachycardia, atrial depolarisation lags behind depolarisation of the ventricles, and inverted P waves may follow the T wave and precede the next QRS complex.

Clinical presentation

Episodes of atrioventricular nodal re-entrant tachycardia may begin at any age. They tend to start and stop abruptly and can occur spontaneously or be precipitated by simple movements. They can

> **Symptoms are commonest in patients with a very rapid heart rate and pre-existing heart disease**

last a few seconds, several hours, or days. The frequency of episodes can vary between several a day, or one episode in a lifetime. Most patients have only mild symptoms, such as palpitations or the sensation that their heart is beating rapidly. More severe symptoms include dizziness, dyspnoea, weakness, neck pulsation, and central chest pain. Some patients report polyuria.

Atrioventricular re-entrant tachycardia

Atrioventricular re-entrant tachycardias occur as a result of an anatomically distinct atrioventricular connection. This accessory conduction pathway allows the atrial impulse to bypass the atrioventricular node and activate the ventricles prematurely (ventricular pre-excitation). The presence of the accessory pathway allows a re-entry circuit to form and paroxysmal atrioventricular re-entrant tachycardias to occur.

> **The commonest kind of atrioventricular re-entrant tachycardia occurs as part of the Wolff-Parkinson-White syndrome**

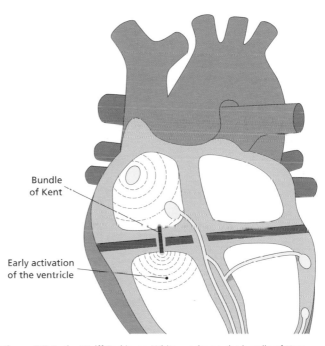

Bundle of Kent

Early activation of the ventricle

Figure 5.5 In the Wolff-Parkinson-White syndrome the bundle of Kent provides a separate electrical conduit between the atria and the ventricles.

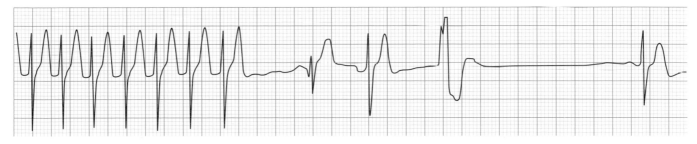

Figure 5.4 Termination of atrioventricular nodal re-entrant tachycardia.

Wolff-Parkinson-White syndrome

In this syndrome an accessory pathway (the bundle of Kent) connects the atria directly to the ventricles. It results from a failure of complete separation of the atria and ventricles during fetal development.

The pathway can be situated anywhere around the groove between the atria and ventricles, and in 10% of cases more than one accessory pathway exists. The accessory pathway allows the formation of a re-entry circuit, which may give rise to either a narrow or a broad complex tachycardia, depending on whether the atrioventricular node or the accessory pathway is used for antegrade conduction.

Electrocardiographic features

In sinus rhythm the atrial impulse conducts over the accessory pathway without the delay encountered with atrioventricular nodal conduction. It is transmitted rapidly to the ventricular myocardium, and consequently the PR interval is short. However, because the impulse enters non-specialised myocardium, ventricular depolarisation progresses slowly at first, distorting the early part of the R wave and producing the characteristic delta wave on the electrocardiogram. This slow depolarisation is then rapidly overtaken by depolarisation propagated by the normal conduction system, and the rest of the QRS complex appears relatively normal.

Commonly, the accessory pathway is concealed—that is, it is capable of conducting only in a retrograde fashion, from ventricles to atria. During sinus rhythm pre-excitation does not occur and the electrocardiogram is normal.

Traditionally the Wolff-Parkinson-White syndrome has been classified into two types according to the electrocardiographic morphology of the precordial leads. In type A, the delta wave and QRS complex are predominantly upright in the precordial leads.

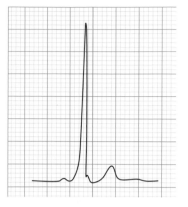

Figure 5.6 In sinus rhythm conduction over the accessory pathway gives rise to a short PR interval and a delta wave.

Table 5.1 Classification of Wolff-Parkinson-White syndrome.

Type A (dominant R wave in V1 lead) may be confused with:
- Right bundle branch block
- Right ventricular hypertrophy
- Posterior myocardial infarction

Type B (negative QRS complex in V1 lead) may be confused with:
- Left bundle branch block
- Anterior myocardial infarction

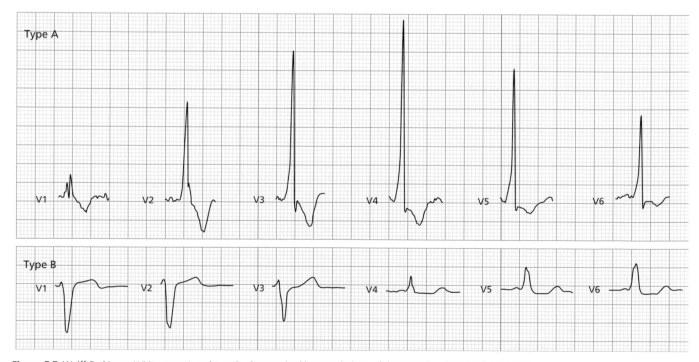

Figure 5.7 Wolff-Parkinson-White, type A and type B, characterised by morphology of the recording from leads V1 to V6.

The dominant R wave in lead V1 may be misinterpreted as right bundle branch block. In type B, the delta wave and QRS complex are predominantly negative in leads V1 and V2 and positive in the other precordial leads, resembling left bundle branch block.

Mechanism of tachycardia formation

Orthodromic atrioventricular re-entrant tachycardias account for most tachycardias in the Wolff-Parkinson-White syndrome. A premature atrial impulse is conducted down the atrioventricular node to the ventricles and then in a retrograde fashion via the accessory pathway back to the atria. The impulse then circles repeatedly between the atria and ventricles, producing a narrow complex tachycardia. Since atrial depolarisation lags behind ventricular depolarisation, P waves follow the QRS complexes. The delta wave is not observed during the tachycardia, and the QRS complex is of normal duration. The rate is usually 140-250 beats/min.

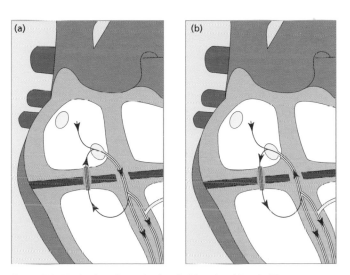

Figure 5.8 Mechanisms for orthodromic (a) and antidromic (b) atrioventricular re-entrant tachycardia.

Antidromic atrioventricular re-entrant tachycardia is relatively uncommon, occurring in about 10% of patients with the Wolff-Parkinson-White syndrome. The accessory pathway allows antegrade conduction, and thus the impulse is conducted from the atria to the ventricles via the accessory pathway. Depolarisation is propagated through non-specialised myocardium, and the resulting QRS complex is broad and bizarre. The impulse then travels in a retrograde fashion via the atrioventricular node back to the atria.

Atrial fibrillation

In patients without an accessory pathway the atrioventricular node protects the ventricles from the rapid atrial activity that occurs during atrial fibrillation. In the Wolff-Parkinson-White syndrome the atrial impulses can be conducted via the accessory pathway,

> *Orthodromic* atrioventricular re-entrant tachycardia occurs with antegrade conduction through the atrioventricular node
>
> *Antidromic* atrioventricular re-entrant tachycardia occurs with retrograde conduction through the atrioventricular node

> In some patients the accessory pathway allows very rapid conduction, and consequently very fast ventricular rates (in excess of 300 beats/min) may be seen, with the associated risk of deterioration into ventricular fibrillation.

causing ventricular pre-excitation and producing broad QRS complexes with delta waves. Occasionally an impulse will be conducted via the atrioventricular node and produce a normal QRS complex. The electrocardiogram has a characteristic appearance, showing a rapid, completely irregular broad complex tachycardia but with occasional narrow complexes.

Clinical presentation

The Wolff-Parkinson-White syndrome is sometimes an incidental electrocardiographic finding, but often patients present with

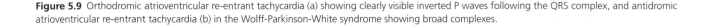

Figure 5.9 Orthodromic atrioventricular re-entrant tachycardia (a) showing clearly visible inverted P waves following the QRS complex, and antidromic atrioventricular re-entrant tachycardia (b) in the Wolff-Parkinson-White syndrome showing broad complexes.

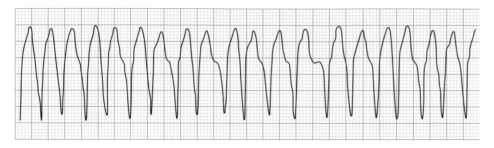

Figure 5.10 Atrial fibrillation in the Wolff-Parkinson-White syndrome.

tachyarrhythmias. Episodes tend to be more common in young people but may come and go through life. Patients may first present when they are old.

When rapid arrhythmias occur in association with atrial fibrillation, patients may present with heart failure or hypotension. Drugs that block the atrioventricular node—for example, digoxin, verapamil, and adenosine—may be dangerous in this situation and should be avoided. These drugs decrease the refractoriness of accessory connections and increase the frequency of conduction, resulting in a rapid ventricular response, which may precipitate ventricular fibrillation.

CHAPTER 6

Broad Complex Tachycardia—Part I

June Edhouse, Francis Morris

Broad complex tachycardias occur by various mechanisms and may be ventricular or supraventricular in origin. In the emergency setting most broad complex tachycardias have a ventricular origin. However, an arrhythmia arising from the atria or the atrioventricular junction will produce a broad complex if associated with ventricular pre-excitation or bundle branch block. The causes of ventricular and supraventricular tachycardias are generally quite different, with widely differing prognoses. Most importantly, the treatment of a broad complex tachycardia depends on the origin of the tachycardia. This chapter describes monomorphic ventricular tachycardias; other ventricular tachycardias and supraventricular tachycardias will be described in the next article.

Terminology

Ventricular tachycardia is defined as three or more ventricular extrasystoles in succession at a rate of more than 120 beats/min. The tachycardia may be self terminating but is described as "sustained" if it lasts longer than 30 seconds. The term "accelerated idioventricular rhythm" refers to ventricular rhythms with rates of 100-120 beats/min.

> Ventricular tachycardia is described as "monomorphic" when the QRS complexes have the same general appearance, and "polymorphic" if there is wide beat to beat variation in QRS morphology. Monomorphic ventricular tachycardia is the commonest form of sustained ventricular tachycardia

Mechanisms of ventricular arrhythmias

The mechanisms responsible for ventricular tachycardia include re-entry or increased myocardial automaticity. The tachycardia is usually initiated by an extrasystole and involves two pathways of conduction with differing electrical properties. The re-entry circuits that support ventricular tachycardia can be "micro" or "macro" in scale and often occur in the zone of ischaemia or fibrosis surrounding damaged myocardium.

Ventricular tachycardia may result from direct damage to the myocardium secondary to ischaemia or cardiomyopathy, or from

Table 6.1 Varieties of broad complex tachycardia.

Ventricular
Regular
- Monomorphic ventricular tachycardia
- Fascicular tachycardia
- Right ventricular outflow tract tachycardia

Irregular
- Torsades de pointes tachycardia
- Polymorphic ventricular tachycardia

Supraventricular
- Bundle branch block with aberrant conduction
- Atrial tachycardia with pre excitation

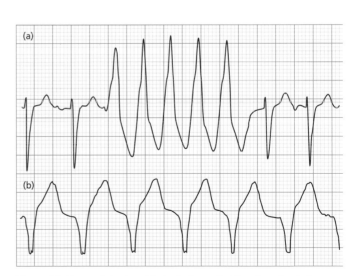

Figure 6.1 Non-sustained ventricular tachycardia (a) and accelerated idioventricular rhythm (b).

> The electrophysiology of a re-entry circuit was described in the previous chapter

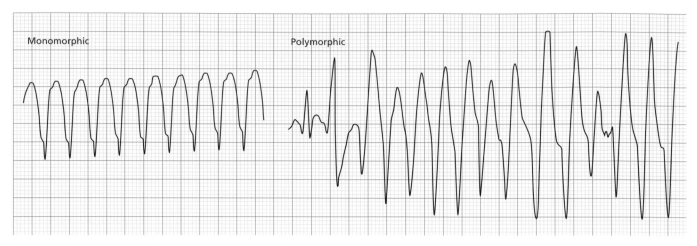

Figure 6.2 Monomorphic and polymorphic ventricular tachycardia.

the effects of myocarditis or drugs—for example, class 1 antiarrhythmics (such as flecainide, quinidine, and disopyramide). Monomorphic ventricular tachycardia usually occurs after myocardial infarction and is a sign of extensive myocardial damage; there is a high in-hospital mortality, more often resulting from impaired ventricular function than recurrence of the arrhythmia.

Electrocardiographic findings in monomorphic ventricular tachycardia

Electrocardiographic diagnosis of monomorphic ventricular tachycardia is based on the following features.

Duration and morphology of QRS complex

In ventricular tachycardia the sequence of cardiac activation is altered, and the impulse no longer follows the normal intraventricular conduction pathway. As a consequence, the morphology of the QRS complex is bizarre, and the duration of the complex is prolonged (usually to 0.12 s or longer).

As a general rule the broader the QRS complex, the more likely the rhythm is to be ventricular in origin, especially if the complexes are greater than 0.16 s. Duration of the QRS complex may exceed 0.2 s, particularly if the patient has electrolyte abnormalities or severe myocardial disease or is taking antiarrhythmic drugs, such as flecainide. If the tachycardia originates in the proximal part of the His-Purkinje system, however, duration can be relatively short—as in a fascicular tachycardia, where QRS duration ranges from 0.11 s to 0.14 s.

The QRS complex in ventricular tachycardia often has a right or left bundle branch morphology. In general, a tachycardia originating in the left ventricle produces a right bundle branch block pattern, whereas a tachycardia originating in the right ventricle results in a left bundle branch block pattern. The intraventricular septum is the focus of the arrhythmia in some patients with ischaemic heart disease, and the resulting complexes have a left bundle branch block morphology.

Rate and rhythm

In ventricular tachycardia the rate is normally 120-300 beats/ minute. The rhythm is regular or almost regular (<0.04 s beat to

> **Triggered automaticity of a group of cells can result from congenital or acquired heart disease. Once initiated, these tachycardias tend to accelerate but slow markedly before stopping**

> **Ventricular tachycardia in a patient with chronic ischaemic heart disease is probably caused by a re-entry phenomenon involving infarct scar tissue, and thus the arrhythmia tends to be recurrent**

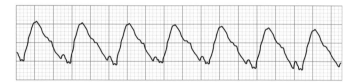

Figure 6.3 Ventricular tachycardia with very broad QRS complexes.

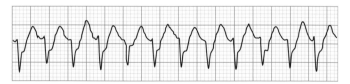

Figure 6.4 Fascicular tachycardia with narrow QRS complexes.

beat variation), unless disturbed by the presence of capture or fusion beats (see below). If a monomorphic broad complex tachycardia has an obviously irregular rhythm the most likely diagnosis is atrial fibrillation with either aberrant conduction or pre-excitation.

Frontal plane axis

In a normal electrocardiogram the QRS axis in the mean frontal plane is between −30° and +90°, with the axis most commonly lying at around 60°. With the onset of ventricular tachycardia the mean frontal plane axis changes from that seen in sinus rhythm and is often bizarre. A change in axis of more than 40° to the left or right is suggestive of ventricular tachycardia.

Lead aVR is situated in the frontal plane at −210°, and when the cardiac axis is normal the QRS complex in this lead is negative; a positive QRS complex in aVR indicates an extremely abnormal axis either to the left or right. When the QRS complex in lead aVR is entirely positive the tachycardia originates close to the apex of the ventricle, with the wave of depolarisation moving upwards towards the base of the heart.

> In some patients the atrioventricular node allows retrograde conduction of ventricular impulses to the atria. The resulting P waves are inverted and occur after the QRS complex, usually with a constant RP interval.

Direct evidence of independent atrial activity

In ventricular tachycardia, the sinus node continues to initiate atrial contraction. Since this atrial contraction is completely independent of ventricular activity, the resulting P waves are dissociated from the QRS complexes and are positive in leads I and II. The atrial rate is usually slower than the ventricular rate, though occasionally 1:1 conduction occurs.

> It is important to scrutinise the tracings from all 12 leads of the electrocardiogram, as P waves may be evident in some leads but not in others

Although evidence of atrioventricular dissociation is diagnostic for ventricular tachycardia, a lack of direct evidence of independent P wave activity does not exclude the diagnosis. The situation may be complicated by artefacts that simulate P wave activity.

However, beat to beat differences, especially of the ST segment, suggest the possibility of independent P wave activity, even though it may be impossible to pinpoint the independent P wave accurately.

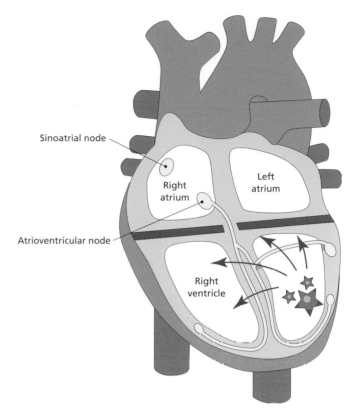

Figure 6.5 Ventricular tachycardia showing abnormal direction of wave of depolarisation, giving rise to bizarre axis.

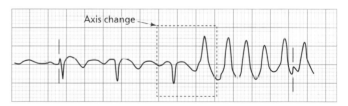

Figure 6.6 Change in axis with onset of monomorphic ventricular tachycardia in lead aVR.

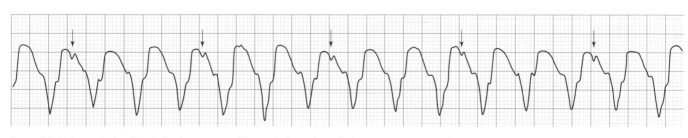

Figure 6.7 Atrioventricular dissociation in monomorphic ventricular tachycardia (note P waves, arrowed).

Indirect evidence of independent atrial activity

Capture beat

Occasionally an atrial impulse may cause ventricular depolarisation via the normal conduction system. The resulting QRS complex occurs earlier than expected and is narrow. Such a beat shows that even at rapid rates the conduction system is able to conduct normally, thus making a diagnosis of supraventricular tachycardia with aberrancy unlikely.

Capture beats are uncommon, and though they confirm a diagnosis of ventricular tachycardia, their absence does not exclude the diagnosis.

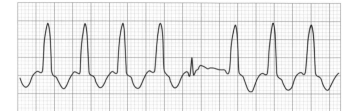

Figure 6.8 Capture beat.

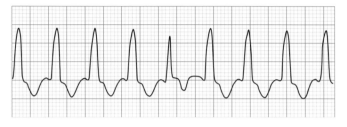

Figure 6.9 Fusion beat.

Fusion beats

A fusion beat occurs when a sinus beat conducts to the ventricles via the atrioventricular node and fuses with a beat arising in the ventricles. As the ventricles are depolarised partly by the impulse conducted through the His-Purkinje system and partly by the impulse arising in the ventricle, the resulting QRS complex has an appearance intermediate between a normal beat and a tachycardia beat.

Like capture beats, fusion beats are uncommon, and though they support a diagnosis of ventricular tachycardia, their absence does not exclude the diagnosis.

QRS concordance throughout the chest leads

Concordance exists when all the QRS complexes in the chest leads are either predominantly positive or predominantly negative.

The presence of concordance suggests that the tachycardia has a ventricular origin.

Positive concordance probably indicates that the origin of the tachycardia lies on the posterior ventricular wall; the wave of depolarisation moves towards all the chest leads and produces positive complexes. Similarly, negative concordance is thought to correlate with a tachycardia originating in the anterior ventricular wall.

Concordance can be either positive or negative

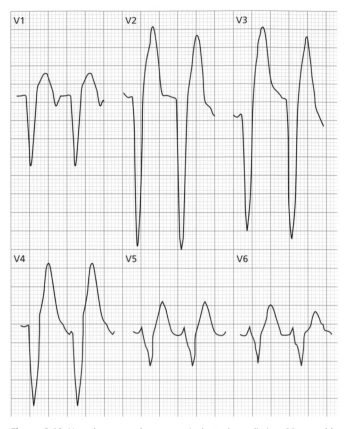

Figure 6.10 Negative concordance: ventricular tachycardia in a 90 year old woman in congestive cardiac failure.

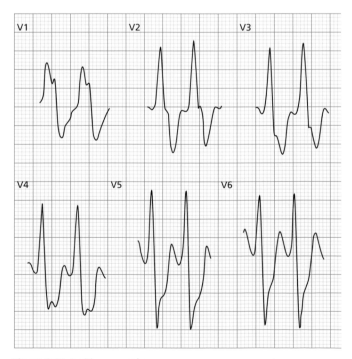

Figure 6.11 Positive concordance.

CHAPTER 7

Broad Complex Tachycardia—Part II

June Edhouse, Francis Morris

This chapter continues the discussion on ventricular tachycardias and also examines how to determine whether a broad complex tachycardia is ventricular or supraventricular in origin.

Ventricular tachycardias

Fascicular tachycardia

Fascicular tachycardia is uncommon and not usually associated with underlying structural heart disease. It originates from the region of the posterior fascicle (or occasionally the anterior fascicle) of the left bundle branch and is partly propagated by the His-Purkinje network. It therefore produces QRS complexes of relatively short duration (0.11-0.14 s). Consequently, this arrhythmia is commonly misdiagnosed as a supraventricular tachycardia.

The QRS complexes have a right bundle branch block pattern, often with a small Q wave rather than primary R wave in lead V1 and a deep S wave in lead V6. When the tachycardia originates from the posterior fascicle the frontal plane axis of the QRS complex is deviated to the left; when it originates from the anterior fascicle, right axis deviation is seen.

Right ventricular outflow tract tachycardia

This tachycardia originates from the right ventricular outflow tract, and the impulse spreads inferiorly. The electrocardiogram typically shows right axis deviation, with a left bundle branch block pattern. The tachycardia may be brief and self terminating or sustained, and it may be provoked by catecholamine release, sudden changes in heart rate, and exercise. The tachycardia usually responds to drugs such as β blockers or calcium antagonists. Occasionally the arrhythmia stops with adenosine treatment and so may be misdiagnosed as a supraventricular tachycardia.

Torsades de pointes tachycardia

Torsades de pointes ("twisting of points") is a type of polymorphic ventricular tachycardia in which the cardiac axis rotates over a sequence of 5-20 beats, changing from one direction to another and back again. The QRS amplitude varies similarly, such that the complexes appear to twist around the baseline. In sinus rhythm the QT interval is prolonged and prominent U waves may be seen.

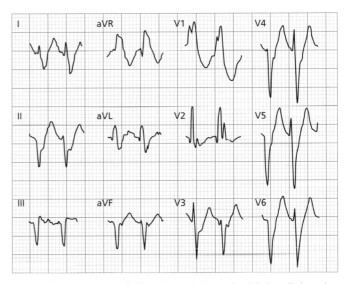

Figure 7.1 Fascicular ventricular tachycardia (note the right bundle branch block pattern and left axis deviation).

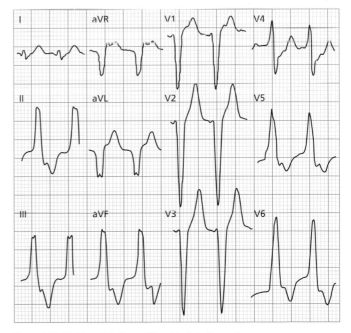

Figure 7.2 Right ventricular outflow track tachycardia.

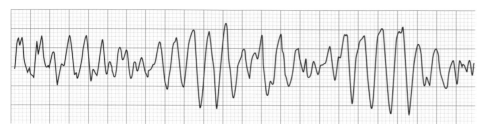

Figure 7.3 Torsades de pointes.

Torsades de pointes is not usually sustained, but it will recur unless the underlying cause is corrected. Occasionally it may be prolonged or degenerate into ventricular fibrillation. It is associated with conditions that prolong the QT interval.

Transient prolongation of the QT interval is often seen in the acute phase of myocardial infarction, and this may lead to torsades de pointes. Ability to recognise torsades de pointes is important because its management is different from the management of other ventricular tachycardias.

Polymorphic ventricular tachycardia

Polymorphic ventricular tachycardia has the electrocardiographic characteristics of torsades de pointes but in sinus rhythm the QT interval is normal. It is much less common than torsades de pointes. If sustained, polymorphic ventricular tachycardia often leads to haemodynamic collapse. It can occur in acute myocardial infarction and may deteriorate into ventricular fibrillation. Polymorphic ventricular tachycardia must be differentiated from atrial fibrillation with pre-excitation, as both have the appearance of an irregular broad complex tachycardia with variable QRS morphology (see Chapter 6).

> **Torsades de pointes may be drug induced or secondary to electrolyte disturbances**

Table 7.1 Causes of torsades de pointes.

Drugs
- Antiarrhythmic drugs: class Ia (disopyramide, procainamide, quinidine); class III (amiodarone, bretylium, sotalol)
- Antibacterials: erythromycin, fluoquinolones, trimethoprim
- Other drugs: terfenadine, cisapride, tricyclic antidepressants, haloperidol, lithium, phenothiazines, chloroquine, thioridazine

Electrolyte disturbances
- Hypokalaemia
- Hypomagnesaemia

Congenital syndromes
- Jervell and Lange-Nielsen syndrome
- Romano-Ward syndrome

Other causes
- Ischaemic heart disease
- Myxoedema
- Bradycardia due to sick sinus syndrome or complete heart block
- Subarachnoid haemorrhage

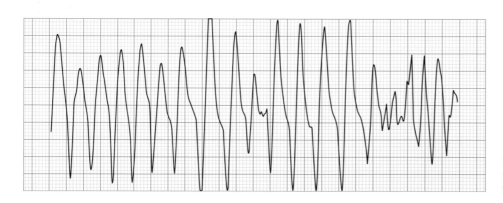

Figure 7.4 Polymorphic ventricular tachycardia deteriorating into ventricular fibrillation.

Broad complex tachycardias of supraventricular origin

In the presence of aberrant conduction or ventricular pre-excitation, any supraventricular tachycardia may present as a broad complex tachycardia and mimic ventricular tachycardia.

Atrial tachycardia with aberrant conduction

Aberrant conduction is defined as conduction through the atrioventricular node with delay or block, resulting in a broader

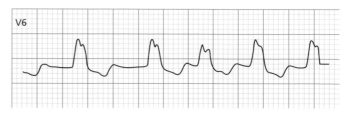

Figure 7.5 Atrial fibrillation and left bundle branch block.

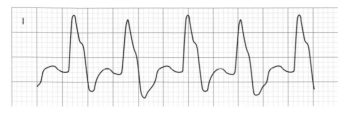

Figure 7.6 Atrial flutter with left bundle branch block, giving rise to broad complex tachycardia.

QRS complex. Aberrant conduction usually manifests as left or right bundle branch block, both of which have characteristic features. The bundle branch block may predate the tachycardia, or it may be a rate related functional block, occurring when atrial impulses arrive too rapidly for a bundle branch to conduct normally. When atrial fibrillation occurs with aberrant conduction and a rapid ventricular response, a totally irregular broad complex tachycardia is produced.

Wolff-Parkinson-White syndrome

Broad complex tachycardias may also occur in the Wolff-Parkinson-White syndrome, either as an antidromic atrioventricular re-entrant tachycardia or in association with atrial flutter or fibrillation.

Antidromic atrioventricular re-entrant tachycardia

In this relatively uncommon tachycardia the impulse is conducted from the atria to the ventricles via the accessory pathway. The resulting tachycardia has broad, bizarre QRS complexes.

Atrial fibrillation

In patients without an accessory pathway the atrioventricular node protects the ventricles from the rapid atrial activity that occurs during atrial fibrillation. In the Wolff-Parkinson-White syndrome the atrial impulses are conducted down the accessory pathway, which may allow rapid conduction and consequently very fast ventricular rates.

The impulses conducted via the accessory pathway produce broad QRS complexes. Occasionally an impulse will be conducted via the atrioventricular node and produce a normal QRS complex or a fusion beat. The result is a completely irregular and often rapid broad complex tachycardia with a fairly constant QRS pattern, except for occasional normal complexes and fusion beats.

Table 7.2 Differentiation between ventricular tachycardia and supraventricular tachycardia with bundle branch block.

If the tachycardia has a right bundle branch block morphology (a predominantly positive QRS complex in lead V1), a ventricular origin is suggested if there is:
- QRS complex with duration >0.14 s
- Axis deviation
- A QS wave or predominantly negative complex in lead V6
- Concordance throughout the chest leads, with all deflections positive
- A single (R) or biphasic (QR or RS) R wave in lead V1
- A triphasic R wave in lead V1, with the initial R wave taller than the secondary R wave and an S wave that passes through the isoelectric line

If the tachycardia has a left bundle branch block morphology (a predominantly negative deflection in lead V1), a ventricular origin is suggested if there is:
- Axis deviation
- QRS complexes with duration >0.16 s
- A QS or predominantly negative deflection in lead V6
- Concordance throughout the chest leads, with all deflections negative
- An rS complex in lead V1

The Wolff-Parkinson-White syndrome is discussed in more detail in an earlier Chapter 5, on junctional tachycardias

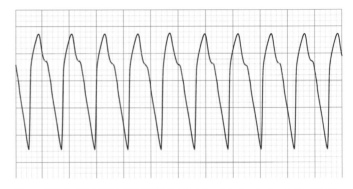

Figure 7.7 Antidromic atrioventricular re-entrant tachycardia, giving rise to broad complex tachycardia.

Drugs that block the atrioventricular node—such as digoxin, verapamil, and adenosine—should be avoided as they can produce an extremely rapid ventricular response

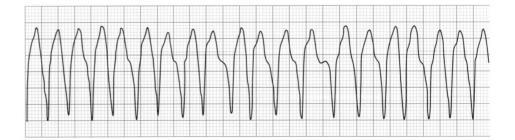

Figure 7.8 Atrial fibrillation in patient with Wolff-Parkinson-White syndrome (note irregularity of complexes).

Differentiating between ventricular and supraventricular origin

Clinical presentation

Age is a useful factor in determining the origin of a broad complex tachycardia: a tachycardia in patients aged over 35 years is more likely to be ventricular in origin. A history that includes ischaemic heart disease or congestive cardiac failure is 90% predictive of ventricular tachycardia.

The symptoms associated with broad complex tachycardia depend on the haemodynamic consequences of the arrhythmia—that is, they relate to the heart rate and the underlying cardiac reserve rather than to the origin of the arrhythmia. It is wrong to assume that a patient with ventricular tachycardia will inevitably be in a state of collapse; some patients look well but present with dizziness, palpitations, syncope, chest pain, or heart failure. In contrast, a supraventricular tachycardia may cause collapse in a patient with underlying poor ventricular function.

Clinical evidence of atrioventricular dissociation—that is, "cannon" waves in the jugular venous pulse or variable intensity of the first heart sound—indicates a diagnosis of a ventricular tachycardia. The absence of these findings, however, does not exclude the diagnosis.

Electrocardiographic differences

Direct evidence of independent P wave activity is highly suggestive of ventricular tachycardia, as is the presence of fusion beats or

Table 7.3 Danger of misdiagnosis.

- The safest option is to regard a broad complex tachycardia of uncertain origin as ventricular tachycardia unless good evidence suggests a supraventricular origin
- If a ventricular tachycardia is wrongly treated as supraventricular tachycardia, the consequences may be extremely serious
- Giving verapamil to a patient with ventricular tachycardia may result in hypotension, acceleration of the tachycardia, and death

In ventricular tachycardia the rhythm is regular or almost regular; if the rhythm is obviously irregular the most likely diagnosis is atrial fibrillation with either aberrant conduction or pre-excitation

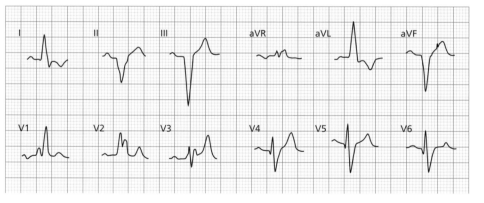

Figure 7.9 Left axis deviation and right bundle branch block in man with previous inferior myocardial infarction.

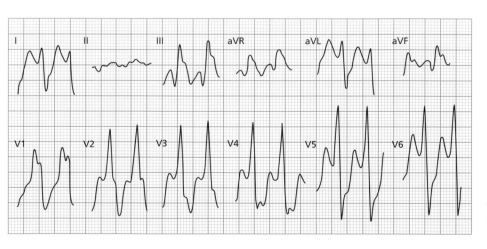

Figure 7.10 Monomorphic ventricular tachycardia in same patient, showing a shift of axis to right of >40° (note positive concordance).

captured beats. The duration of QRS complexes is also a key differentiating feature: those of >0.14 s generally indicate a ventricular origin. Concordance throughout the chest leads also indicates ventricular tachycardia.

A previous electrocardiogram may give valuable information. Evidence of a myocardial infarction increases the likelihood of ventricular tachycardia, and if the mean frontal plane axis changes during the tachycardia (especially if the change is $>40°$ to the left or right) this points to a ventricular origin.

Ventricular tachycardia and supraventricular tachycardia with bundle branch block may produce similar electrocardiograms. If a previous electrocardiogram shows a bundle branch block pattern during sinus rhythm that is similar to or identical with that during the tachycardia, the origin of the tachycardia is likely to be supraventricular. But if the QRS morphology changes during the tachycardia, a ventricular origin is indicated.

Adenosine can also be used to block conduction temporarily through the atrioventricular node to ascertain the origin of a broad complex tachycardia, but failure to stop the tachycardia does not necessarily indicate a ventricular origin

The emergency management of a broad complex tachycardia depends on the wellbeing of the patient and the origin of the arrhythmia. Vagal stimulation—for example, carotid sinus massage or the Valsalva manoeuvre—does not usually affect a ventricular tachycardia but may affect arrhythmias of supraventricular origin. By transiently slowing or blocking conduction through the atrioventricular node, an atrioventricular nodal re-entrant tachycardia or atrioventricular re-entrant tachycardia may be terminated. In atrial flutter transient block may reveal the underlying flutter waves.

CHAPTER 8

Acute Myocardial Infarction—Part I

Francis Morris, William J Brady

In the clinical assessment of chest pain, electrocardiography is an essential adjunct to the clinical history and physical examination. A rapid and accurate diagnosis in patients with acute myocardial infarction is vital, as expeditious reperfusion therapy can improve prognosis. The most frequently used electrocardiographic criterion for identifying acute myocardial infarction is ST segment elevation in two or more anatomically contiguous leads. The ST segment elevation associated with an evolving myocardial infarction is often readily identifiable, but a knowledge of the common "pseudo" infarct patterns is essential to avoid the unnecessary use of thrombolytic treatment.

In the early stages of acute myocardial infarction the electrocardiogram may be normal or near normal; less than half of patients with acute myocardial infarction have clear diagnostic changes on their first trace. About 10% of patients with a proved acute myocardial infarction (on the basis of clinical history and enzymatic markers) fail to develop ST segment elevation or depression. In most cases, however, serial electrocardiograms show evolving changes that tend to follow well recognised patterns.

Hyperacute T waves

The earliest signs of acute myocardial infarction are subtle and include increased T wave amplitude over the affected area. T waves become more prominent, symmetrical, and pointed ("hyperacute"). Hyperacute T waves are most evident in the anterior chest leads and are more readily visible when an old electrocardiogram is available for comparison. These changes in T waves are usually present for only five to 30 minutes after the onset of the infarction and are followed by ST segment changes.

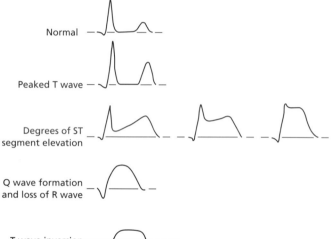

Figure 8.1 Sequence of changes seen during evolution of myocardial infarction.

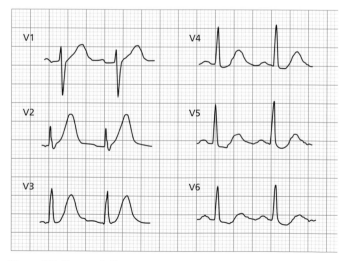

Figure 8.2 Hyperacute T waves.

Table 8.1 Indications for thrombolytic treatment.

- ST elevation >1 mm in two contiguous limb leads or >2 mm in two contiguous chest leads
- Posterior myocardial infarction
- Left bundle branch block

ST segment depression or enzymatic change are not indications for thrombolytic treatment

Sometimes the QRS complex, the ST segment, and the T wave fuse to form a single monophasic deflection, called a giant R wave or "tombstone"

ST segment changes

In practice, ST segment elevation is often the earliest recognised sign of acute myocardial infarction and is usually evident within hours of the onset of symptoms. Initially the ST segment may straighten, with loss of the ST-T wave angle. Then the T wave becomes broad and the ST segment elevates, losing its normal concavity. As further elevation occurs, the ST segment tends to become convex upwards. The degree of ST segment elevation varies between subtle changes of < 1 mm to gross elevation of > 10 mm.

Pathological Q waves

As the acute myocardial infarction evolves, changes to the QRS complex include loss of R wave height and the development of pathological Q waves.

Both of these changes develop as a result of the loss of viable myocardium beneath the recording electrode, and the Q waves are the only firm electrocardiographic evidence of myocardial necrosis. Q waves may develop within one to two hours of the onset of symptoms of acute myocardial infarction, though often they take 12 hours and occasionally up to 24 hours to appear. The presence of pathological Q waves, however, does not necessarily indicate a completed infarct. If ST segment elevation and Q waves are evident on the electrocardiogram and the chest pain is of recent onset, the patient may still benefit from thrombolysis or direct intervention.

When there is extensive myocardial infarction, Q waves act as a permanent marker of necrosis. With more localised infarction the scar tissue may contract during the healing process, reducing the size of the electrically inert area and causing the disappearance of the Q waves.

Resolution of changes in ST segment and T waves

As the infarct evolves, the ST segment elevation diminishes and the T waves begin to invert. The ST segment elevation associated with an inferior myocardial infarction may take up to two weeks to resolve. ST segment elevation associated with anterior myocardial infarction may persist for even longer, and if a left ventricular aneurysm develops it may persist indefinitely. T wave inversion may also persist for many months and occasionally remains as a permanent sign of infarction.

Reciprocal ST segment depression

ST segment depression in leads remote from the site of an acute infarct is known as reciprocal change and is a highly sensitive indicator of acute myocardial infarction. Reciprocal changes are seen in up to 70% of inferior and 30% of anterior infarctions.

Typically, the depressed ST segments tend to be horizontal or downsloping. The presence of reciprocal change is particularly useful when there is doubt about the clinical significance of ST segment elevation.

Reciprocal change strongly indicates acute infarction, with a sensitivity and positive predictive value of over 90%, though its absence does not rule out the diagnosis.

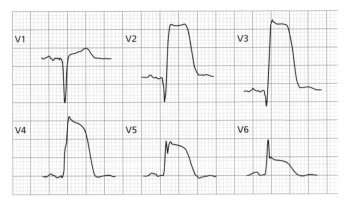

Figure 8.3 Anterior myocardial infarction with gross ST segment elevation (showing "tombstone" R waves).

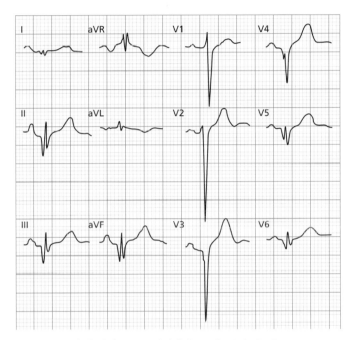

Figure 8.4 Pathological Q waves in inferior and anterior leads.

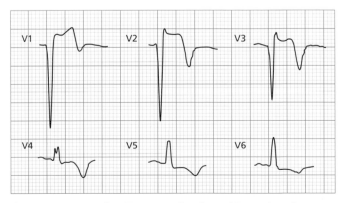

Figure 8.5 Long standing ST segment elevation and T wave inversion associated with a previous anterior myocardial infarction (echocardiography showed a left ventricular aneurysm).

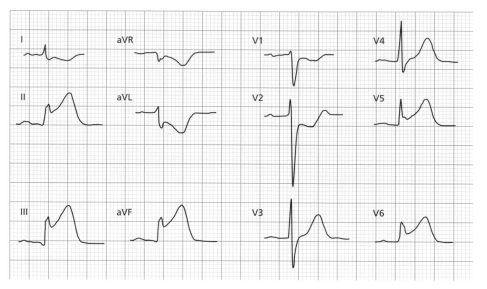

Figure 8.6 An inferolateral myocardial infarction with reciprocal changes in leads I, aVL, V1, and V2.

The pathogenesis of reciprocal change is uncertain. Reciprocal changes are most frequently seen when the infarct is large, and they may reflect an extension of the infarct or occur as a result of coexisting remote ischaemia. Alternatively, it may be a benign electrical phenomenon. The positive potentials that are recorded by electrodes facing the area of acute injury are projected as negative deflections in leads opposite the injured area, thus producing a "mirror image" change. Extensive reciprocal ST segment depression in remote regions often indicates widespread arterial disease and consequently carries a worse prognosis.

Table 8.2 Anatomical relationship of lead.

Inferior wall—Leads II, III, and aVF
Anterior wall—Leads V1 to V4
Lateral wall—Leads I, aVL, V5, and V6

Non-standard leads
Right ventricle—Right sided chest leads V1R to V6R
Posterior wall—Leads V7 to V9

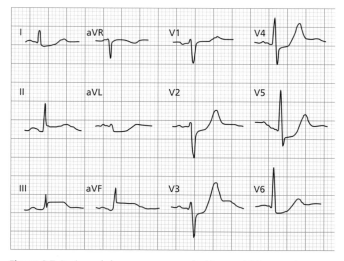

Figure 8.7 Reciprocal changes: presence of widespread ST segment depression in the anterolateral leads strongly suggests that the subtle inferior ST segment elevation is due to acute infarction.

Localisation of site of infarction

The distribution of changes recorded in acute myocardial infarction allows the area of infarction to be localised, thus indicating the site of arterial disease. Proximal arterial occlusions tend to produce the most widespread electrocardiographic abnormalities. The anterior and inferior aspects of the heart are the areas most commonly subject to infarction. Anteroseptal infarcts are highly specific indicators of disease of the left anterior descending artery. Isolated inferior infarcts—changes in leads II, III, and aVF—are usually associated with disease in the right coronary or distal circumflex artery. Disease in the proximal circumflex artery is often associated with a lateral infarct pattern—that is, in leads I, aVL, V5, and V6.

Right ventricular infarction

Right ventricular infarction is often overlooked, as standard 12 lead electrocardiography is not a particularly sensitive indicator of right ventricular damage. Right ventricular infarction is associated with 40% of inferior infarctions. It may also complicate some anterior infarctions but rarely occurs as an isolated phenomenon. On the standard 12 lead electrocardiogram right ventricular infarction is indicated by signs of inferior infarction, associated with ST segment elevation in lead V1. It is unusual for ST segment elevation in lead V1 to occur as an isolated phenomenon.

Right sided chest leads are much more sensitive to the presence of right ventricular infarction. The most useful lead is lead V4R (an electrode is placed over the right fifth intercostal space in the midclavicular line). Lead V4R should be recorded as soon as possible

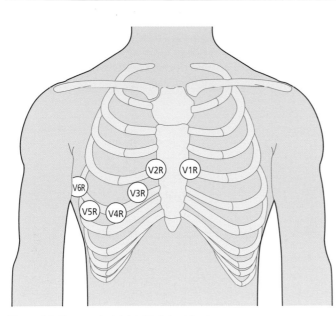

Figure 8.8 Placement of right sided chest leads.

in all patients with inferior infarction, as ST segment elevation in right ventricular infarction may be short lived.

Right ventricular infarction usually results from occlusion of the right coronary artery proximal to the right ventricular marginal branches, hence its association with inferior infarction. Less commonly, right ventricular infarction is associated with occlusion of the circumflex artery, and if this vessel is dominant there may be an associated inferolateral wall infarction.

Posterior myocardial infarction

Posterior myocardial infarction refers to infarction of the posterobasal wall of the left ventricle. The diagnosis is often missed as the standard 12 lead electrocardiography does not include posterior leads. Early detection is important as expeditious thrombolytic treatment may improve the outcome for patients with posterior infarction.

The changes of posterior myocardial infarction are seen indirectly in the anterior precordial leads. Leads V1 to V3 face the endocardial surface of the posterior wall of the left ventricle. As these leads record from the opposite side of the heart instead of

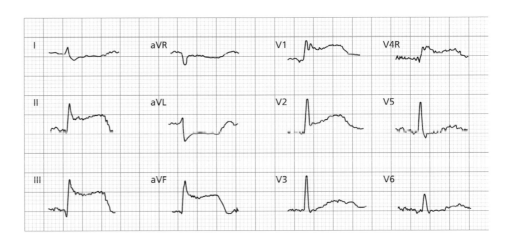

Figure 8.9 Acute inferior myocardial infarction with associated right ventricular infarction.

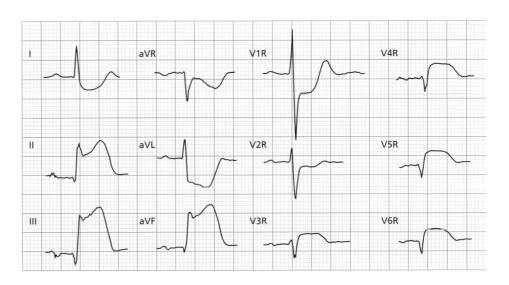

Figure 8.10 Acute inferior myocardial infarction with right ventricular involvement.

directly over the infarct, the changes of posterior infarction are reversed in these leads. The R waves increase in size, becoming broader and dominant, and are associated with ST depression and upright T waves. This contrasts with the Q waves, ST segment elevation, and T wave inversion seen in acute anterior myocardial infarction. Ischaemia of the anterior wall of the left ventricle also produces ST segment depression in leads V1 to V3, and this must be differentiated from posterior myocardial infarction. The use of posterior leads V7 to V9 will show ST segment elevation in patients with posterior infarction. These additional leads therefore provide valuable information, and they help in identfying the patients who may benefit from urgent reperfusion therapy.

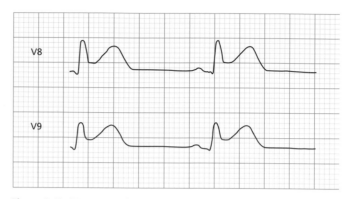

The diagnosis of right ventricular infarction is important as it may be associated with hypotension. Treatment with nitrates or diuretics may compound the hypotension, though the patient may respond to a fluid challenge

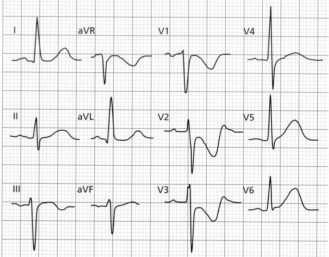

Figure 8.12 ST segment elevation in posterior chest leads V8 and V9.

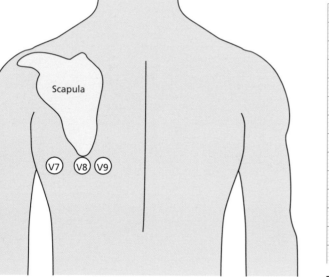

Figure 8.11 Position of V7, V8, and V9 on posterior chest wall.

Figure 8.13 Isolated posterior infarction with no associated inferior changes (note ST segment depression in leads V1 to V3).

CHAPTER 9

Acute Myocardial Infarction—Part II

June Edhouse, William J Brady, Francis Morris

This chapter describes the association of bundle branch block with acute myocardial infarction and the differential diagnosis of ST segment elevation.

Bundle branch block

Acute myocardial infarction in the presence of bundle branch block carries a much worse prognosis than acute myocardial infarction with normal ventricular conduction. This is true both for patients whose bundle branch block precedes the infarction and for those in whom bundle branch block develops as a result of the acute event. Thrombolytic treatment produces dramatic reductions in mortality in these patients, and the greatest benefits are seen in those treated early. It is therefore essential that the electrocardiographic identification of acute myocardial infarction in patients with bundle branch block is both timely and accurate.

Left bundle branch block

Left bundle branch block is most commonly seen in patients with coronary artery disease, hypertension, or dilated cardiomyopathy. The left bundle branch usually receives blood from the left anterior descending branch of the left coronary artery and from the right coronary artery. When new left bundle branch block occurs in the context of an acute myocardial infarction the infarct is usually anterior and mortality is extremely high.

The electrocardiographic changes of acute myocardial infarction can be difficult to recognise when left bundle branch block is present, and many of the conventional diagnostic criteria are not applicable.

Abnormal ventricular depolarisation in left bundle branch block leads to secondary alteration in the recovery process (see earlier chapter about bradycardias and atrioventricular conduction block). This appears on the electrocardiogram as repolarisation changes in a direction opposite to that of the main QRS deflection—that is, "appropriate discordance" between the QRS complex and the ST segment.

Thus leads with a predominantly negative QRS complex show ST segment elevation with positive T waves (an appearance similar to that of acute anterior myocardial infarction).

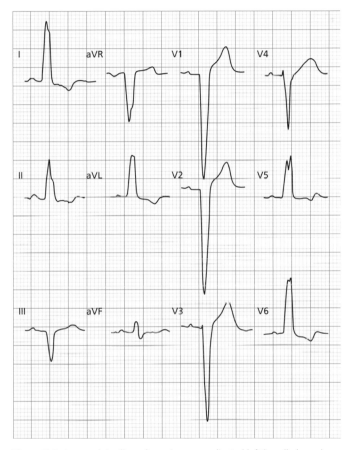

Figure 9.1 Appropriate discordance in uncomplicated left bundle branch block (note ST elevation in leads V1 to V3).

Recognition of acute ischaemia

Many different electrocardiographic criteria have been proposed for identifying acute infarction in left bundle branch block, but none has yet proved sufficiently sensitive to be useful in the acute setting. However, some features are specific indicators of acute ischaemia.

ST segment elevation in association with a positive QRS complex, or ST segment depression in leads V1, V2, or V3 (which have predominantly negative QRS complexes), is not expected in uncomplicated left bundle branch block and is termed "inappropriate concordance."

Inappropriate concordance strongly indicates acute ischaemia. Extreme ST segment elevation (≥5 mm) in leads V1 and V2 also suggests acute ischaemia. If doubt persists, serial electrocardiograms may show evolving changes.

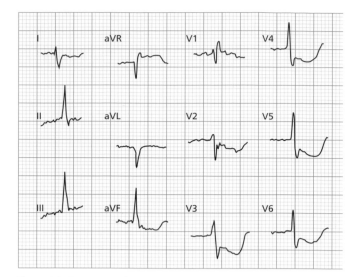

Figure 9.3 ST segment depression in precordial leads in 68 year old man with chest pain.

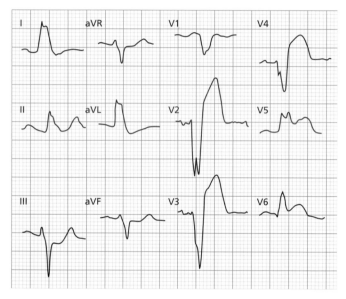

Figure 9.2 Acute myocardial infarction and left bundle branch block. Note that the ST segments are elevated in leads V5 and V6 (inappropriate concordance) and grossly elevated (>5 mm) in leads V2, V3, and V4; note also the ST segment depression in leads III and aVF.

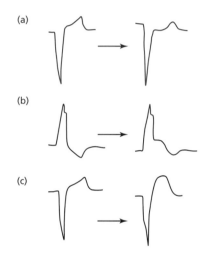

Figure 9.4 Inappropriate concordance in lead V1 in patient with left bundle branch block (a); inappropriate concordance in lead V6 in patient with left bundle branch block (b); and exaggeration of appropriate discordance in lead V1 in patient with left bundle branch block (c).

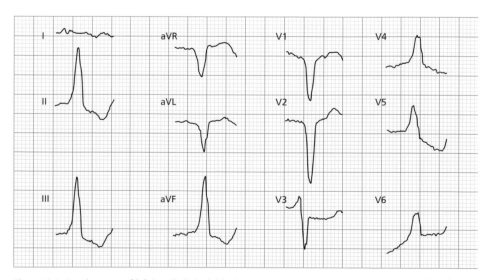

Figure 9.5 Development of left bundle branch block in same man shown in Figure 9.3 shortly after admission (note ST segment depression in lead V3; this is an example of inappropriate concordance).

Right bundle branch block

Right bundle branch block is most commonly seen in association with coronary artery disease, but in many cases no organic heart disease is present. Uncomplicated right bundle branch block usually causes little ST segment displacement and neither causes nor masks Q waves. Thus it does not generally interfere with the diagnosis of acute myocardial infarction, though it may mask a posterior myocardial infarction.

Differential diagnosis of ST segment elevation

ST segment elevation has numerous possible causes. It may be a variant of normal or be due to cardiac or non-cardiac disease. A correct diagnosis has obvious advantages for the patient but is also particularly important before the use of thrombolytic treatment so that unnecessary exposure to the risks of thrombolytic drugs can be avoided.

The interpretation of ST segment elevation should always be made in the light of the clinical history and examination findings. There are often clues in the electrocardiogram to differentiate the ST segment elevation of acute ischaemia from other causes; for example, reciprocal changes (see Chapter 8) may be present, which strongly indicate acute ischaemia.

Serial electrocardiography or continuous ST segment monitoring is also useful as ischaemic ST segment elevation evolves over time. Old electrocardiograms are also useful for comparison.

"High take-off"

Care is required when interpreting ST segment elevation in right sided chest leads as the ST segments, particularly in leads V2 and V3, tend to be upsloping rather than flat. Isolated ST segment elevation in these leads should be interpreted with caution. (For more information on "high take-off" see Chapter 2.)

Benign early repolarisation

A degree of ST segment elevation is often present in healthy individuals, especially in young adults and in people of African descent. This ST segment elevation is most commonly seen in the precordial leads and is often most marked in lead V4. It is usually subtle but can sometimes be pronounced and can easily be mistaken for pathological ST segment elevation.

Benign early repolarisation can be recognised by its characteristic electrocardiographic features: elevation of the J point above the isoelectric line, with high take-off of the ST segment; a distinct notch at the junction of the R wave and S wave, the J point; an upward concavity of the ST segment; and symmetrical, upright T waves, often of large amplitude.

Antecedent myocardial infarction

The ST segment elevation associated with acute infarction usually resolves within two weeks of the acute event, but it may persist indefinitely, especially when associated with anterior myocardial infarction. In these patients a diagnosis of left ventricular aneurysm should be considered. Care should be taken when interpreting the electrocardiogram within two weeks of an acute event, and comparison with old electrocardiograms may be useful.

> The Brugada syndrome, which is familial, occurs particularly in young men and is characterised by right bundle branch block and ST segment elevation in the right precordial leads. There is a high instance of death as a result of ventricular tachyarrhythmias

Table 9.1 Causes of ST segment elevation.

- Acute myocardial infarction
- "High take-off"
- Benign early repolarisation
- Left bundle branch block
- Left ventricular hypertrophy
- Ventricular aneurysm
- Coronary vasospasm/Printzmetal's angina
- Pericarditis
- Brugada syndrome
- Subarachnoid haemorrhage

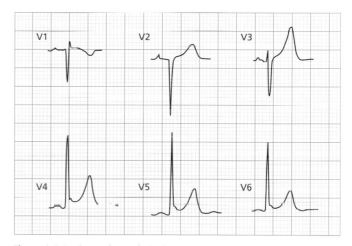

Figure 9.6 Benign early repolarisation.

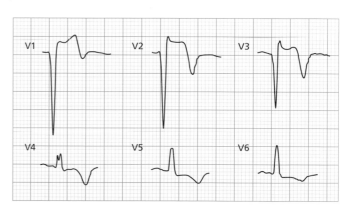

Figure 9.7 Persistent ST segment elevation in anterior chest leads in association with left ventricular aneurysm.

Acute pericarditis

Acute pericarditis is commonly mistaken for acute myocardial infarction as both cause chest pain and ST segment elevation. In pericarditis, however, the ST segment elevation is diffuse rather than localised, often being present in all leads except aVR and V1. The elevated ST segments are concave upwards, rather than convex upwards as seen in acute infarction. Depression of the PR segment may also be seen.

ST segment elevation in pericarditis is thought to be due to the associated subepicardial myocarditis. The zone of injured tissue causes abnormal ST vectors; the end result is that leads facing the epicardial surface record ST segment elevation, whereas those facing the ventricular cavity (leads aVR and V1) record ST segment depression. The absence of widespread reciprocal change, the presence of PR segment depression, and absence of Q waves may be helpful in distinguishing pericarditis from acute myocardial infarction.

Other causes of ST segment elevation

The characteristic features of left ventricular hypertrophy are also often misinterpreted as being caused by acute ischaemia. ST segment elevation in the precordial leads is a feature of left ventricular hypertrophy and is due to secondary repolarisation abnormalities.

ST segment abnormalities are seen in association with intracranial (particularly subarachnoid) haemorrhage. ST segment elevation or depression may be seen; a putative explanation is that altered autonomic tone affects the duration of ventricular repolarisation, producing these changes.

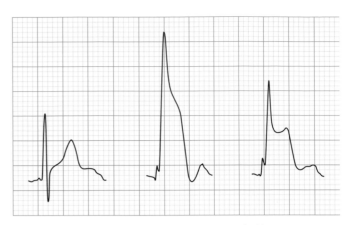

Figure 9.9 Reversible ST segment elevation associated with coronary artery spasm.

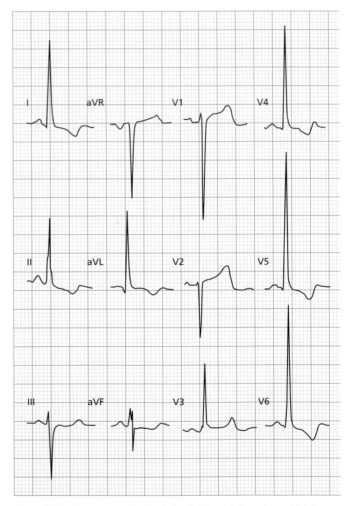

Figure 9.10 ST segment elevation in leads V1 to V3 in patient with left ventricular hypertrophy.

Printzmetal's angina (vasospastic angina) is associated with ST segment elevation. As the changes are due to coronary artery spasm rather than acute infarction, they may be completely reversible if treated promptly. ST segment abnormalities may be seen in association with cocaine use and are probably due to a combination of vasospasm and thrombosis.

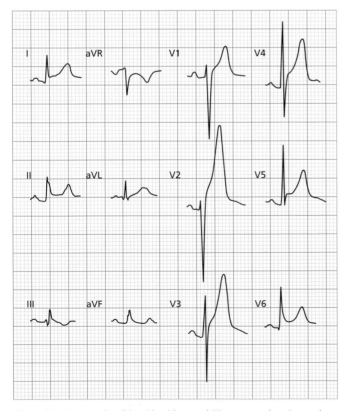

Figure 9.8 Acute pericarditis with widespread ST segment elevation and PR segment depression (see lead II).

CHAPTER 10

Myocardial Ischaemia

Kevin Channer, Francis Morris

In clinical practice electrocardiography is most often used to evaluate patients with suspected ischaemic heart disease. When interpreted in the light of the clinical history, electrocardiograms can be invaluable in aiding selection of the most appropriate management.

Electrocardiography has limitations. A trace can suggest, for example, that a patient's heart is entirely normal when in fact he or she has severe and widespread coronary artery disease. In addition, less than half of patients presenting to hospital with an acute myocardial infarction will have the typical and diagnostic electrocardiographic changes present on their initial trace, and as many as 20% of patients will have a normal or near normal electrocardiogram.

Myocardial ischaemia causes changes in the ST-T wave, but unlike a full thickness myocardial infarction it has no direct effects on the QRS complex (although ischaemia may give rise to bundle branch blocks, which prolongs the QRS complex).

When electrocardiographic abnormalities occur in association with chest pain but in the absence of frank infarction, they confer prognostic significance. About 20% of patients with ST segment depression and 15% with T wave inversion will experience severe angina, myocardial infarction, or death within 12 months of their initial presentation, compared with 10% of patients with a normal trace.

Changes in the ST segment and T waves are not specific for ischaemia; they also occur in association with several other disease processes, such as left ventricular hypertrophy, hypokalaemia, and digoxin therapy.

T wave changes

Myocardial ischaemia can affect T wave morphology in a variety of ways: T waves may become tall, flattened, inverted, or biphasic. Tall T waves are one of the earliest changes seen in acute myocardial infarction, most often seen in the anterior chest leads. Isolated tall T waves in leads V1 to V3 may also be due to ischaemia of the posterior wall of the left ventricle (the mirror image of T wave inversion).

As there are other causes of abnormally tall T waves and no commonly used criteria for the size of T waves, these changes are not always readily appreciated without comparison with a previous electrocardiogram. Flattened T waves are often seen in patients with myocardial ischaemia, but they are very non-specific.

Electrocardiography is not sufficiently specific or sensitive to be used without a patient's clinical history

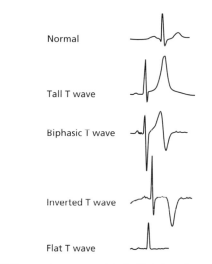

Normal

Tall T wave

Biphasic T wave

Inverted T wave

Flat T wave

Figure 10.1 T wave changes associated with ischaemia.

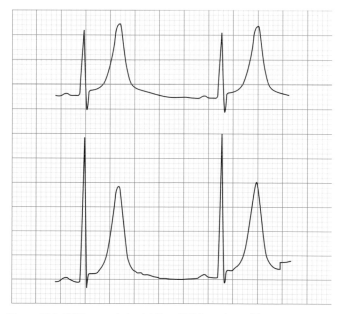

Figure 10.2 Tall T waves in leads V2 and V3 in patient with recent inferoposterior myocardial infarction, indicating posterior ischaemia.

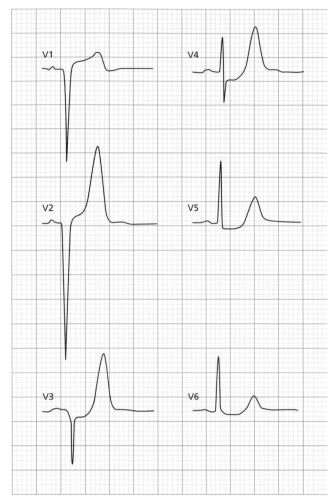

Figure 10.3 Tall T waves in myocardial ischaemia.

Myocardial ischaemia may also give rise to T wave inversion, but it must be remembered that inverted T waves are normal in leads III, aVR, and V1 in association with a predominantly negative QRS complex. T waves that are deep and symmetrically inverted (arrowhead) strongly suggest myocardial ischaemia.

In some patients with partial thickness ischaemia the T waves show a biphasic pattern. This occurs particularly in the anterior chest leads and is an acute phenomenon. Biphasic T wave changes usually evolve and are often followed by symmetrical T wave inversion. These changes occur in patients with unstable or crescendo angina and strongly suggest myocardial ischaemia.

Table 10.1 Suggested criteria for size of T wave.

- 1/8 size of the R wave
- <2/3 size of the R wave
- Height <10 mm

Table 10.2 T wave inversion.

- T wave inversion can be normal
- It occurs in leads III, aVR, and V1 (and in V2, but only in association with T wave inversion in lead V1)

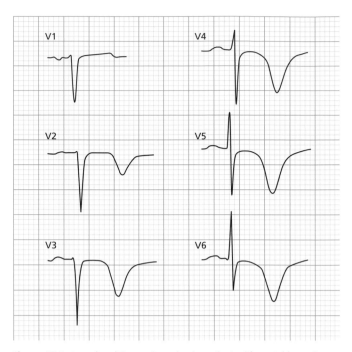

Figure 10.4 Arrowhead T wave inversion in patient with unstable angina.

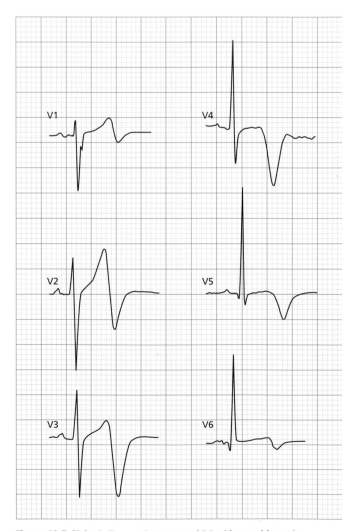

Figure 10.5 Biphasic T waves in man aged 26 with unstable angina.

ST segment depression

Typically, myocardial ischaemia gives rise to ST segment depression. The normal ST segment usually blends with the T wave smoothly, making it difficult to determine where the ST segment ends and the T wave starts. One of the first and most subtle changes in the ST segment is flattening of the segment, resulting in a more obvious angle between the ST segment and T wave.

More obvious changes comprise ST segment depression that is usually planar (horizontal) or downsloping. Whereas horizontal ST depression strongly suggests ischaemia, downsloping changes are less specific as they are also found in association with left ventricular hypertrophy and in patients taking digoxin. The degree of ST segment depression in any given lead is related to the size of the R wave. Thus, ST segment depression is usually most obvious in leads V4 to V6 of the 12 lead electrocardiogram. Moreover, because the height of the R wave varies with respiration, the degree of ST depression in any one lead may vary from beat to beat. ST segment depression is usually not as marked in the inferior leads because here the R waves tend to be smaller. Substantial (≥2 mm) and

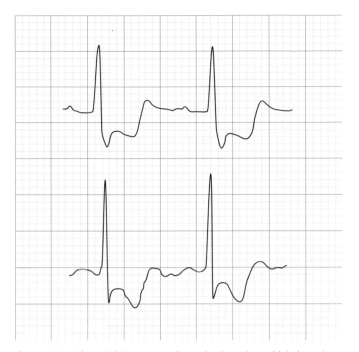

Figure 10.8 Substantial ST segment depression in patient with ischaemic chest pain (diagram is scaled up).

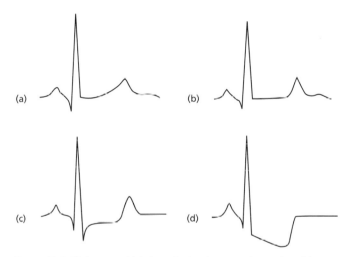

Figure 10.6 ST changes with ischaemia showing normal wave form (a); flattening of ST segment (b), making T wave more obvious; horizontal (planar) ST segment depression (c); and downsloping ST segment depression (d).

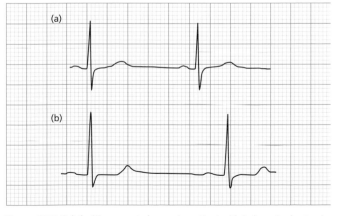

Figure 10.7 Subtle ST segment change in patient with ischaemic chest pain: when no pain is present (a) and when in pain (b).

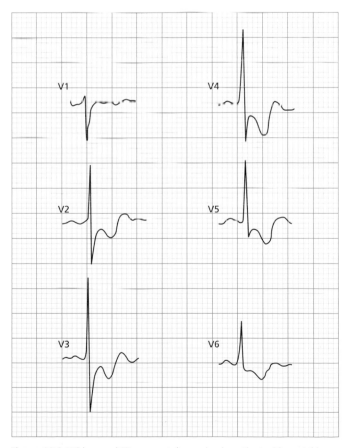

Figure 10.9 Widespread ST segment depression in patient with unstable angina (diagram is scaled up).

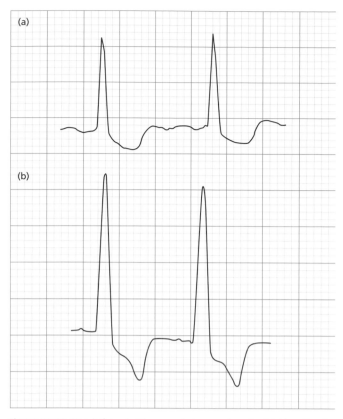

Figure 10.10 Non-ischaemic ST segment changes: in patient taking digoxin (a) and in patient with left ventricular hypertrophy (b).

widespread (≥2 leads) ST depression is a grave prognostic finding as it implies widespread myocardial ischaemia from extensive coronary artery disease. ST segment depression may be transient, and its resolution with treatment is reassuring. Modern equipment allows continuous ST segment monitoring. Serial changes in the electrocardiogram over a few hours or days, especially when the changes are associated with recurrent chest pain, are extremely helpful in confirming the presence of ischaemic heart disease; serial changes confer a worse prognosis, indicating the need for increased drug treatment or revascularisation interventions.

ST segment elevation

Transient ST segment elevation in patients with chest pain is a feature of ischaemia and is usually seen in vasospastic (variant or Prinzmetal's) angina. A proportion of these patients, however, will have substantial proximal coronary artery stenosis. When ST segment elevation has occurred and resolved it may be followed by deep T wave inversion even in the absence of enzyme evidence of myocardial damage.

In patients with previous Q wave myocardial infarction the hallmark of new ischaemia is often ST segment elevation. This is thought to be associated with a wall motion abnormality, or bulging of the infarcted segment. It rarely indicates reinfarction in the same territory. When an electrocardiogram shows persistent T wave inversion accompanying the changes of a previous acute myocardial infarction, ischaemia in the same territory may cause

"normalisation" of the T waves (return to an upright position). Alternatively, further ischaemia may make the T wave inversion more pronounced.

Arrhythmias associated with acute myocardial ischaemia or infarction

Ventricular myocardial ischaemia may be arrhythmogenic, and extrasystoles are common. It used to be thought that frequent extrasystoles of multifocal origin, bigeminy, couplets, or extrasystoles that fell on the T wave (R on T) conferred a bad prognosis in the early hours of myocardial infarction and predicted the onset of ventricular fibrillation. Clinical trials have clearly shown, however, that their suppression by antiarrhythmic drugs had no effect on the frequency of subsequent ventricular fibrillation.

Ventricular fibrillation is the commonest unheralded fatal arrhythmia in the first 24 hours of acute myocardial infarction.

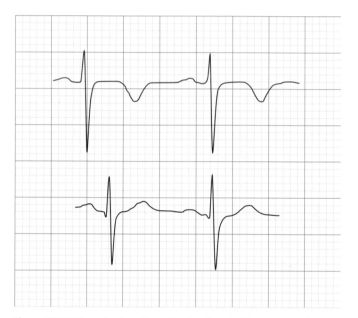

Figure 10.11 Normalisation of longstanding inverted T waves in patient with chest pain.

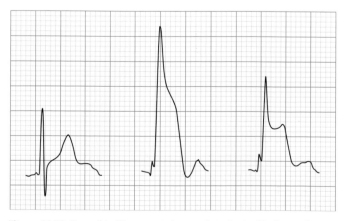

Figure 10.12 Reversible ST segment changes in patient with chest pain; the ST segment elevation returns to normal as the chest pain settles.

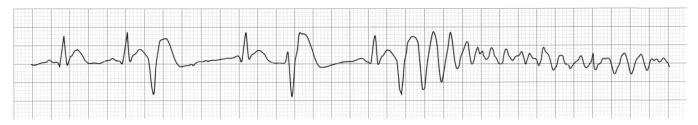

Figure 10.13 R on T, giving rise to ventricular fibrillation.

The prognosis depends almost entirely on the patient's proximity to skilled medical help when the arrhythmia occurs. Cardiac arrest from ventricular fibrillation outside hospital is associated with a long term survival of about 10%, compared with an initial survival of 90% when cardiac arrest occurs after admission to a coronary care unit. Studies have shown that the key factor in prognosis is the speed with which electrical defibrillation is delivered.

Heart block

The artery supplying the atrioventricular node is usually a branch of the right coronary artery; less commonly it originates from the left circumflex artery. In patients with proximal occlusion of the right coronary artery causing an inferior infarction, the atrioventricular node's arterial supply may be compromised resulting in various degrees of heart block. Atrioventricular block may be severe at first but usually improves over subsequent days. Complete atrioventricular block usually gives way to second degree and then first degree block. Although temporary transvenous cardiac pacing may be necessary for patients who are haemodynamically compromised, it is not mandatory in stable patients.

> **Short runs of ventricular tachycardia are a bad prognostic sign and should probably be treated**

> **Tachycardias of supraventricular origin, with the exception of atrial fibrillation, are uncommon after myocardial infarction. Atrial fibrillation occurs in about 10% of patients and is more common in those with heart failure, diabetes, and valvular heart disease. It may be transient or persistent and is often a marker of haemodynamic instability**

> **When complete atrioventricular block occurs in association with acute anterior myocardial infarction, transvenous cardiac pacing is recommended**

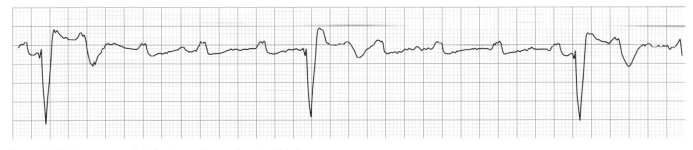

Figure 10.14 Acute myocardial infarction with complete heart block.

Profound bradycardia or atrioventricular block resulting from ischaemia may provoke an escape rhythm. Such rhythms are the result of spontaneous activity from a subsidiary pacemaker located within the atria, atrioventricular junction, or ventricles. An atrioventricular junction escape beat has a normal QRS complex morphology, with a rate of 40-60 beats/min. A ventricular escape rhythm is broad complex and generally slower (15-40 beats/min).

CHAPTER 11

Exercise Tolerance Testing

Jonathan Hill, Adam Timmis

Exercise tolerance testing is an important diagnostic and prognostic tool for assessing patients with suspected or known ischaemic heart disease. During exercise, coronary blood flow must increase to meet the higher metabolic demands of the myocardium. Limiting the coronary blood flow may result in electrocardiographic changes. This chapter reviews the electrocardiographic responses that occur with exercise, both in normal subjects and in those with ischaemic heart disease.

Clinical relevance

Exercise tolerance testing (also known as exercise testing or exercise stress testing) is used routinely in evaluating patients who present with chest pain, in patients who have chest pain on exertion, and in patients with known ischaemic heart disease.

Exercise testing has a sensitivity of 78% and a specificity of 70% for detecting coronary artery disease. It cannot therefore be used to rule in or rule out ischaemic heart disease unless the probability of coronary artery disease is taken into account. For example, in a low risk population, such as men aged under 30 years and women aged under 40, a positive test result is more likely to be a false positive than true, and negative results add little new information. In a high risk population, such as those aged over 50 with typical angina symptoms, a negative result cannot rule out ischaemic heart disease, though the results may be of some prognostic value.

Exercise testing is therefore of greatest diagnostic value in patients with an intermediate risk of coronary artery disease.

The test

Protocol

The Bruce protocol is the most widely adopted protocol and has been extensively validated. The protocol has seven stages, each lasting three minutes, resulting in 21 minutes' exercise for a complete test. In stage 1 the patient walks at 1.7 mph (2.7 km) up a 10% incline. Energy expenditure is estimated to be 4.8 METs (metabolic equivalents) during this stage. The speed and incline increase with each stage. A modified Bruce protocol is used for exercise testing within one week of myocardial infarction.

> **ST segment depression (horizontal or downsloping) is the most reliable indicator of exercise-induced ischaemia**

Table 11.1 Prognostic indications for exercise testing.

- Risk stratification after myocardial infarction
- Risk stratification in patients with hypertrophic cardiomyopathy
- Evaluation of revascularisation or drug treatment
- Evaluation of exercise tolerance and cardiac function
- Assessment of cardiopulmonary function in patients with dilated cardiomyopathy or heart failure
- Assessment of treatment for arrhythmia

Table 11.2 Diagnostic indications for exercise testing.

- Assessment of chest pain in patients with intermediate probability for coronary artery disease
- Arrhythmia provocation
- Assessment of symptoms (for example, presyncope) occurring during or after exercise

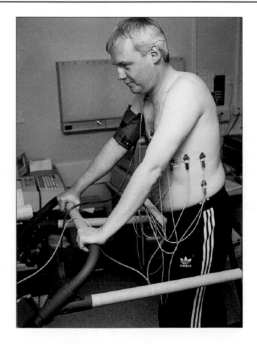

Figure 11.1 Patient exercising on treadmill.

Preparing the patient

β blockers should be discontinued the day before the test, and dixogin (which may cause false positive results, with ST segment abnormalities) should be stopped one week before testing.

The patient is first connected to the exercise electrocardiogram machine. Resting electrocardiograms, both sitting and standing, are recorded as electrocardiographic changes, particularly T wave inversion, may occur as the patient stands up to start walking on the treadmill. A short period of electrocardiographic recording during hyperventilation is also valuable for identifying changes resulting from hyperventilation rather than from coronary ischaemia.

During the test the electrocardiogram machine provides a continuous record of the heart rate, and the 12 lead electrocardiogram is recorded intermittently. Blood pressure must be measured before the exercise begins and at the end of each exercise stage. Blood pressure may fall or remain static during the initial stage of exercise. This is the result of an anxious patient relaxing. As the test progresses, however, systolic blood pressure should rise as exercise increases. A level of up to 225 mm Hg is normal in adults, although athletes can have higher levels. Diastolic blood pressure tends to fall slightly. The aim of the exercise is for the patient to achieve their maximum predicted heart rate.

Safety

If patients are carefully selected for exercise testing, the rate of serious complications (death or acute myocardial infarction) is about 1 in 10 000 tests (0.01%). The incidence of ventricular tachycardia or fibrillation is about 1 in 5000. Full cardiopulmonary resuscitation facilities must be available, and test supervisors must be trained in cardiopulmonary resuscitation.

Limitations

The specificity of ST segment depression as the main indicator of myocardial ischaemia is limited. ST segment depression has been estimated to occur in up to 20% of normal individuals on ambulatory electrocardiographic monitoring. There are many causes of ST segment changes apart from coronary artery disease, which confound the result of exercise testing. If the resting electrocardiogram is abnormal, the usefulness of an exercise test is reduced or may even be precluded. Repolarisation and conduction abnormalities—for example, left ventricular hypertrophy, left bundle branch block, pre-excitation, and effects of digoxin—preclude accurate interpretation of the electrocardiogram during exercise, and as a result, other forms of exercise test (for example, adenosine or dobutamine scintigraphy) or angiography are required to evaluate this group of patients.

Normal trace during exercise

The J point (the point of inflection at the junction of the S wave and ST segment) becomes depressed during exercise, with maximum depression at peak exercise. The normal ST segment during exercise therefore slopes sharply upwards.

By convention, ST segment depression is measured relative to the isoelectric baseline (between the T and P waves) at a point 60-80 ms after the J point. There is intraobserver variation in the

Table 11.3 Workload.

- Assessment of workload is measured by metabolic equivalents (METs)
- Workload is a reflection of oxygen consumption and hence energy use
- 1 MET is 3.5 ml oxygen/kg per minute, which is the oxygen consumption of an average individual at rest
- To carry out the activities of daily living an exercise intensity of at least 5 METs is required

Table 11.4 Maximum predicted heart rate.

- By convention, the maximum predicted heart rate is calculated as 220 (210 for women) minus the patient's age
- A satisfactory heart rate response is achieved on reaching 85% of the maximum predicted heart rate
- Attainment of maximum heart rate is a good prognostic sign

Table 11.5 Contraindications for exercise testing.

- Acute myocardial infarction (within 4-6 days)
- Unstable angina (rest pain in previous 48 hours)
- Uncontrolled heart failure
- Acute myocarditis or pericarditis
- Acute systemic infection
- Deep vein thrombosis
- Uncontrolled hypertension (systolic blood pressure > 220 mm Hg, diastolic > 120 mm Hg)
- Severe aortic stenosis
- Severe hypertrophic obstructive cardiomyopathy
- Untreated life threatening arrhythmia
- Dissecting aneurysm
- Recent aortic surgery

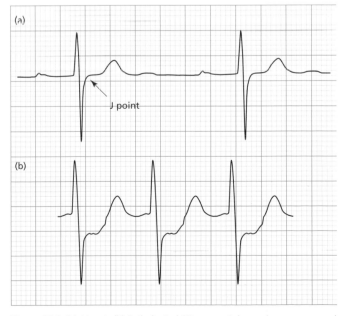

Figure 11.2 (a) At rest. (b) Pathological ST segment depression as measured 80 ms from J point.

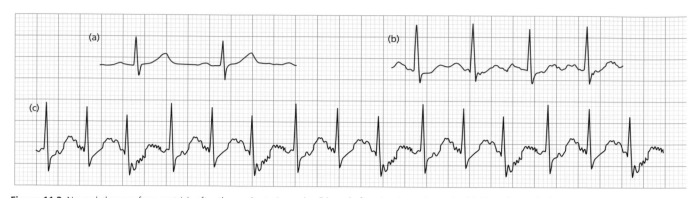

Figure 11.3 Normal changes from rest (a), after three minutes' exercise (b), and after six minutes' exercise (c). Note the upsloping ST segments.

measurement of this ST segment depression, and therefore a computerised analysis that accompanies the exercise test can assist but not replace the clinical evaluation of the test.

Abnormal changes during exercise

The standard criterion for an abnormal ST segment response is horizontal (planar) or downsloping depression of >1 mm. If 0.5 mm of depression is taken as the standard, the sensitivity of the test increases and the specificity decreases (vice versa if 2 mm of depression is selected as the standard).

Other recognised abnormal responses to exercise include ST elevation of >1 mm, particularly in the absence of Q waves.

Table 11.6 Normal electrocardiographic changes during exercise.

- P wave increases in height
- R wave decreases in height
- J point becomes depressed
- ST segment becomes sharply upsloping
- Q-T interval shortens
- T wave decreases in height

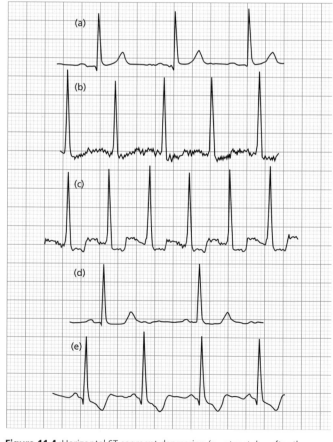

Figure 11.4 Horizontal ST segment depression (a = at rest, b = after three minutes' exercise, c = after six minutes' exercise) and downsloping ST segment depression (d = at rest, e = after six minutes' exercise).

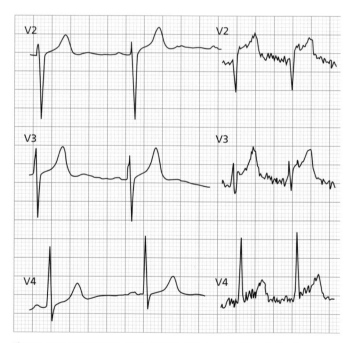

Figure 11.5 ST segments in leads V2 to V4 at rest (left) and after two minutes' exercise (right) (note obvious ST elevation).

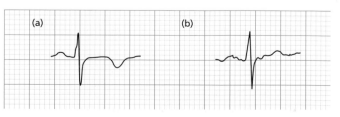

Figure 11.6 T wave inversion in lead V5 at rest (a) and normalisation of T waves with exercise (b).

This suggests severe coronary artery disease and is a sign of poor prognosis. T wave changes such as inversion and pseudo-normalisation (an inverted T wave that becomes upright) are non-specific changes.

A highly specific sign for ischaemia is inversion of the U wave. As U waves are often difficult to identify, especially at high heart rates, this finding is not sensitive. The presence of extrasystoles that have been induced by exercise is neither sensitive nor specific for coronary artery disease.

Stopping the test

In clinical practice, patients rarely exercise for the full duration (21 minutes) of the Bruce protocol. However, completion of 9-12 minutes of exercise or reaching 85% of the maximum predicted changes in heart rate is usually satisfactory. An exercise test should end when diagnostic criteria have been reached or when the patient's symptoms and signs dictate.

After the exercise has stopped, recording continues for up to 15 minutes. ST segment changes (or arrhythmias) may occur during the recovery period that were not apparent during exercise. Such changes generally carry the same significance as those occurring during exercise.

Table 11.7 Reasons for stopping a test.

Electrocardiographic criteria

- Severe ST segment depression (> 3 mm)
- ST segment elevation > 1 mm in non-Q wave lead
- Frequent ventricular extrasystoles (unless the test is to assess ventricular arrhythmia)
- Onset of ventricular tachycardia
- New atrial fibrillation or supraventricular tachycardia
- Development of new bundle branch block (if the test is primarily to detect underlying coronary disease)
- New second or third degree heart block
- Cardiac arrest

Symptoms and signs

- Patient requests stopping because of severe fatigue
- Severe chest pain, dyspnoea, or dizziness
- Fall in systolic blood pressure (> 20 mm Hg)
- Rise in blood pressure (systolic > 300 mm Hg, diastolic > 130 mm Hg)
- Ataxia

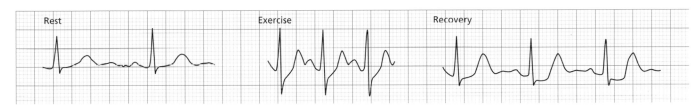

Figure 11.7 Marked ST changes in recovery but not during exercise.

Interpreting the results

Diagnostic testing

Any abnormal electrocardiographic changes must be interpreted in the light of the probability of coronary artery disease and physiological response to exercise. A normal test result or a result that indicates a low probability of coronary artery disease is one in which 85% of the maximum predicted heart rate is achieved with a physiological response in blood pressure and no associated ST segment depression.

A test that indicates a high probability of coronary artery disease is one in which there is substantial ST depression at low work rate associated with typical angina-like pain and a drop in blood pressure. Deeper and more widespread ST depression generally indicates more severe or extensive disease.

False positive results are common in women, reflecting the lower incidence of coronary artery disease in this group.

Prognostic testing

Exercise testing in patients who have just had a myocardial infarction is indicated only in those in whom a revascularisation procedure is contemplated; a less strenuous protocol is used. Testing provides prognostic information. Patients with low

> The most common reason for stopping an exercise test is fatigue and breathlessness as a result of the unaccustomed exercise

Table 11.8 Findings suggesting high probability of coronary artery disease.

- Horizontal ST segment depression of ≤ 2 mm
- Downsloping ST segment depression
- Early positive response within six minutes
- Persistence of ST depression for more than six minutes into recovery
- ST segment depression in five or more leads
- Exertional hypotension

Table 11.9 Rationale for testing.

- Bayes's theorem of diagnostic probability states that the predictive value of an abnormal exercise test will vary according to the probability of coronary artery disease in the population under study
- Exercise testing is therefore usually performed in patients with a moderate probability of coronary artery disease, rather than in those with a very low or high probability

exercise capacity and hypotension induced by exercise have a poor prognosis. Asymptomatic ST segment depression after myocardial infarction is associated with a more than 10-fold increase in mortality compared with a normal exercise test. Conversely, patients who reach stage 3 of a modified Bruce protocol with a blood pressure response of >30 mm Hg have an annual mortality of <2%. Exercise testing can also add prognostic information in patients after percutaneous transluminal coronary angiography or coronary artery bypass graft.

Screening

Exercise testing of asymptomatic patients is controversial because of the high false positive rate in such individuals. Angina remains the most reliable indicator of the need for further investigation.

In certain asymptomatic groups with particular occupations (for example, pilots) there is a role for regular exercise testing, though more stringent criteria for an abnormal test result (such as ST segment depression of >2 mm) should be applied. In the United Kingdom, drivers of heavy goods vehicles and public service vehicles have to achieve test results clearly specified by the Driver and Vehicle Licensing Agency before they are considered fit to drive.

CHAPTER 12

Conditions Affecting the Right Side of the Heart

Richard A Harrigan, Kevin Jones

Many diseases of the right side of the heart are associated with electrocardiographic abnormalities. Electrocardiography is neither a sensitive nor specific tool for diagnosing conditions such as right atrial enlargement, right ventricular hypertrophy, or pulmonary hypertension. However, an awareness of the electrocardiographic abnormalities associated with these conditions may support the patient's clinical assessment and may prevent the changes on the electrocardiogram from being wrongly attributed to other conditions, such as ischaemia.

Right atrial enlargement

The forces generated by right atrial depolarisation are directed anteriorly and inferiorly and produce the early part of the P wave. Right atrial hypertrophy or dilatation is therefore associated with tall P waves in the anterior and inferior leads, though the overall duration of the P wave is not usually prolonged. A tall P wave (height ≥2.5 mm) in leads II, III, and aVF is known as the P pulmonale.

The electrocardiographic changes suggesting right atrial enlargement often correlate poorly with the clinical and pathological findings. Right atrial enlargement is associated with chronic obstructive pulmonary disease, pulmonary hypertension, and congenital heart disease—for example, pulmonary stenosis and tetralogy of Fallot. In practice, most cases of right atrial enlargement are associated with right ventricular hypertrophy, and this may be reflected in the electrocardiogram. The electrocardiographic features of right atrial enlargement without coexisting right ventricular hypertrophy are seen in patients with tricuspid stenosis. P pulmonale may appear transiently in patients with acute pulmonary embolism.

Right ventricular hypertrophy

The forces generated by right ventricular depolarisation are directed rightwards and anteriorly and are almost completely masked by the dominant forces of left ventricular depolarisation. In the presence of right ventricular hypertrophy the forces of depolarisation increase, and if the hypertrophy is severe these forces may dominate on the electrocardiogram.

The electrocardiogram is a relatively insensitive indicator of the presence of right ventricular hypertrophy, and in mild cases of right ventricular hypertrophy the trace will be normal.

This chapter discusses right atrial enlargement, right ventricular hypertrophy, and the electrocardiographic changes associated with chronic obstructive pulmonary disease, pulmonary embolus, acute right heart strain, and valvular heart disease

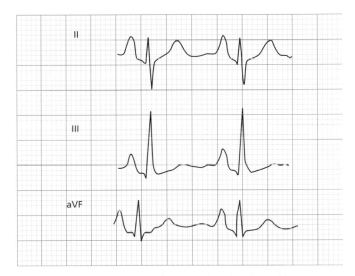

Figure 12.1 Large P waves in leads II, III, and aVF (P pulmonale).

Right ventricular hypertrophy is associated with pulmonary hypertension, mitral stenosis, and less commonly, conditions such as pulmonary stenosis and congenital heart disease

Table 12.1 Diagnostic criteria for right ventricular hypertrophy.

(Provided the QRS duration is less than 0.12 s)
- Right axis deviation of + 110° or more
- Dominant R wave in lead V1
- R wave in lead V1 ≥7 mm

Supporting criteria
- ST segment depression and T wave inversion in leads V1 to V4
- Deep S waves in leads V5, V6, I, and aVL

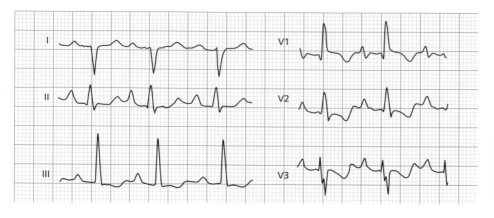

Figure 12.2 Right ventricular hypertrophy secondary to pulmonary stenosis (note the dominant R wave in lead V1, presence of right atrial hypertrophy, right axis deviation, and T wave inversion in leads V1 to V3).

Lead V1 lies closest to the right ventricular myocardium and is therefore best placed to detect the changes of right ventricular hypertrophy, and a dominant R wave in lead V1 is observed. The increased rightward forces are reflected in the limb leads, in the form of right axis deviation. Secondary changes may be observed in the right precordial chest leads, where ST segment depression and T wave inversion are seen.

A dominant R wave in lead V1 can occur in other conditions, but the absence of right axis deviation allows these conditions to be differentiated from right ventricular hypertrophy. Isolated right axis deviation is also associated with a range of conditions.

Chronic obstructive pulmonary disease

In chronic obstructive pulmonary disease, hyperinflation of the lungs leads to depression of the diaphragm, and this is associated with clockwise rotation of the heart along its longitudinal axis. This clockwise rotation means that the transitional zone (defined as the progression of rS to qR in the chest leads) shifts towards the left with persistence of an rS pattern as far as V5 or even V6. This may give rise to a "pseudoinfarct" pattern, with deep S waves in the right precordial leads simulating the appearance of the QS waves and poor R wave progression seen in anterior myocardial infarction. The amplitude of the QRS complexes may be small in patients with chronic obstructive pulmonary disease as the hyperinflated lungs are poor electrical conductors.

Cardiac arrhythmias may occur in patients with chronic obstructive pulmonary disease, particularly in association with an acute

Table 12.2 Conditions associated with tall R wave in lead V1.

- Right ventricular hypertrophy
- Posterior myocardial infarction
- Type A Wolff-Parkinson-White syndrome
- Right bundle branch block

A tall R wave in lead V1 is normal in children and young adults

Table 12.3 Conditions associated with right axis deviation.

- Right ventricular hypertrophy
- Left posterior hemiblock
- Lateral myocardial infarction
- Acute right heart strain

Right axis deviation is normal in infants and children

About three quarters of patients with chronic obstructive pulmonary disease have electrocardiographic abnormalities. P pulmonale is often but not invariably present and may occur with or without clinical evidence of cor pulmonale

In chronic obstructive pulmonary disease the electrocardiographic signs of right ventricular hypertrophy may be present, indicating the presence of cor pulmonale

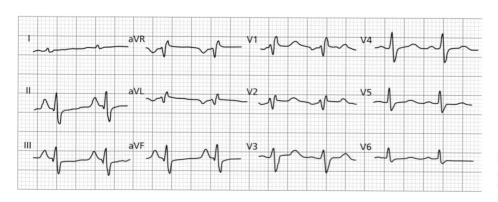

Figure 12.3 Chronic obstructive pulmonary disease (note the P pulmonale, low amplitude QRS complexes, and poor R wave progression).

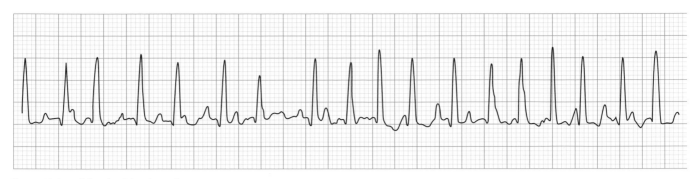

Figure 12.4 Multifocal atrial tachycardia.

respiratory tract infection, respiratory failure, or pulmonary embolism. Arrhythmias are sometimes the result of the underlying disease process but may also occur as side effects of the drugs used to treat the disease.

The arrhythmias are mostly supraventricular in origin and include atrial extrasystoles, atrial fibrillation or flutter, and multifocal atrial tachycardia. Ventricular extrasystoles and ventricular tachycardia may also occur.

Acute pulmonary embolism

The electrocardiographic features of acute pulmonary embolism depend on the size of the embolus and its haemodynamic effects and on the underlying cardiopulmonary reserve of the patient. The timing and frequency of the electrocardiographic recording is also important as changes may be transient. Patients who present with a small pulmonary embolus are likely to have a normal electrocardiogram or a trace showing only sinus tachycardia.

If the embolus is large and associated with pulmonary artery obstruction, acute right ventricular dilatation may occur. This may produce an S wave in lead I and a Q wave in lead III. T wave inversion in lead III may also be present, producing the well known S1, Q3, T3 pattern.

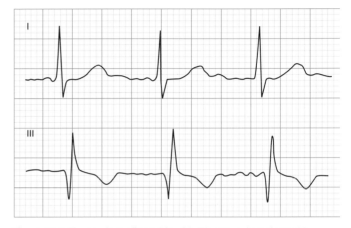

Figure 12.5 Sinus tachycardia and S1, Q3, T3 pattern in patient with pulmonary embolus (diagram scaled up).

The S1, Q3, T3 pattern is seen in about 12% of patients with a massive pulmonary embolus

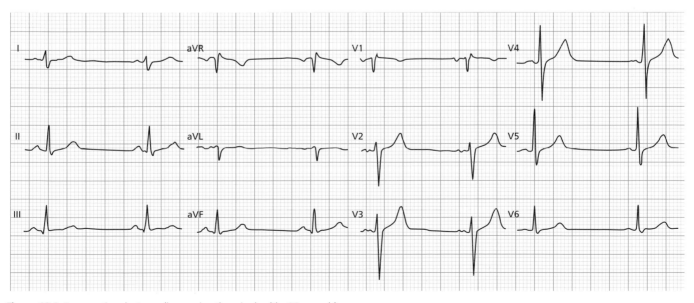

Figure 12.6 Preoperative electrocardiogram in otherwise healthy 38 year old man.

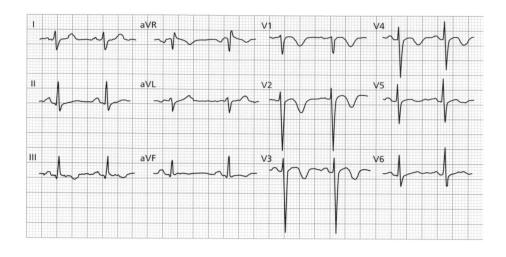

Figure 12.7 Acute pulmonary embolism: 10 days postoperatively the same patient developed acute dyspnoea and hypotension (note the T wave inversion in the right precordial leads and lead III).

Acute right heart strain

When the electrocardiogram shows features of right ventricular hypertrophy accompanied by ST segment depression and T wave inversion, a ventricular "strain" pattern is said to exist. Ventricular strain is seen mainly in leads V1 and V2. The mechanism is unclear. A strain pattern is sometimes seen in acute massive pulmonary embolism but is also seen in patients with right ventricular hypertrophy in the absence of any detectable stress on the ventricle. Both pneumothorax and massive pleural effusion with acute right ventricular dilatation may also produce a strain pattern.

Right sided valvular problems

Tricuspid stenosis

Tricuspid stenosis is a rare disorder and is usually associated with rheumatic heart disease. It appears in the electrocardiogram as P pulmonale. It generally occurs in association with mitral valve disease, and therefore the electrocardiogram often shows evidence of biatrial enlargement, indicated by a large biphasic P wave in

> Right ventricular dilatation may lead to right sided conduction delays, which manifest as incomplete or complete right bundle branch block. There may be some rightward shift of the frontal plane QRS axis. Right atrial dilatation may lead to prominent P waves in the inferior leads. Atrial arrhythmias including flutter and fibrillation are common, and T wave inversion in the right precordial leads may also occur

Table 12.4 Electrocardiographic abnormalities found in acute pulmonary embolism.

- Sinus tachycardia
- Atrial flutter or fibrillation
- S1, Q3, T3 pattern
- Right bundle branch block (incomplete or complete)
- T wave inversion in the right precordial leads
- P pulmonale
- Right axis deviation

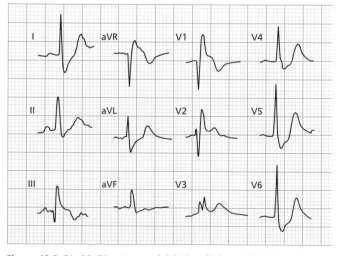

Figure 12.8 S1, Q3, T3 pattern and right bundle branch block in patient with pulmonary embolus.

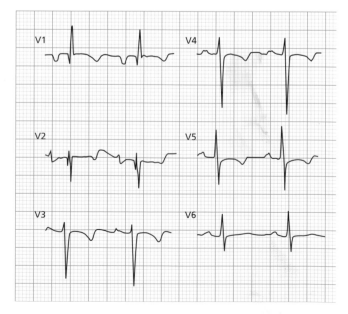

Figure 12.9 Example of right heart strain: right ventricular hypertrophy with widespread T wave inversion in chest leads.

lead V1 with an initial positive deflection followed by a terminal negative deflection.

Tricuspid regurgitation

The electrocardiogram is an unhelpful tool for diagnosing tricuspid regurgitation and generally shows the features of the underlying cardiac disease. The electrocardiographic manifestations of tricuspid regurgitation are non-specific and include incomplete right bundle branch block and atrial fibrillation.

Pulmonary stenosis

Pulmonary stenosis leads to pressure overload in the right atrium and ventricle. The electrocardiogram may be completely normal in the presence of mild pulmonary stenosis. More severe lesions are

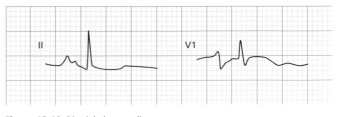

Figure 12.10 Biatrial abnormality.

associated with electrocardiographic features of right atrial and ventricular hypertrophy, with tall P waves, marked right axis deviation, and a tall R wave in lead V1.

CHAPTER 13

Conditions Affecting the Left Side of the Heart

June Edhouse, R K Thakur, Jihad M Khalil

Many cardiac and systemic illnesses can affect the left side of the heart. After a careful history and examination, electrocardiography and chest radiography are first line investigations. Electrocardiography can provide supportive evidence for conditions such as aortic stenosis, hypertension, and mitral stenosis. Recognition of the associated electrocardiographic abnormalities is important as misinterpretation may lead to diagnostic error. This chapter describes the electrocardiographic changes associated with left atrial hypertrophy, left ventricular hypertrophy, valvular disease, and cardiomyopathies.

Left atrial abnormality

The term left atrial abnormality is used to imply the presence of atrial hypertrophy or dilatation, or both. Left atrial depolarisation contributes to the middle and terminal portions of the P wave. The changes of left atrial hypertrophy are therefore seen in the late portion of the P wave. In addition, left atrial depolarisation may be delayed, which may prolong the duration of the P wave.

The P wave in lead V1 is often biphasic. Early right atrial forces are directed anteriorly giving rise to an initial positive deflection; these are followed by left atrial forces travelling posteriorly, producing a later negative deflection. A large negative deflection (> 1 small square in area) suggests a left atrial abnormality. Prolongation of P wave duration to greater than 0.12 s is often found in association with a left atrial abnormality. Normal P waves may be bifid, the minor notch probably resulting from slight asynchrony between right and left atrial depolarisation. However, a pronounced notch with a peak-to-peak interval of > 0.04 s suggests left atrial enlargement.

Any condition causing left ventricular hypertrophy may produce left atrial enlargement as a secondary phenomenon. Left atrial enlargement can occur in association with systemic hypertension, aortic stenosis, mitral incompetence, and hypertrophic cardiomyopathy.

Left ventricular hypertrophy

Systemic hypertension is the most common cause of left ventricular hypertrophy, but others include aortic stenosis and co-arctation of the aorta. Many electrocardiographic criteria have been

Table 13.1 Conditions affecting left side of heart covered in this chapter.

- Left atrial hypertrophy
- Left ventricular hypertrophy
- Valvular disease
- Cardiomyopathies (hypertrophic, dilated, restrictive)

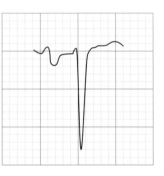

Figure 13.1 Biphasic P wave in V1. The large negative deflection indicates left atrial abnormality (enlarged to show detail).

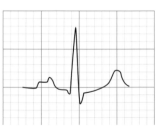

Figure 13.2 P mitrale in lead II. P mitrale is a P wave that is abnormally notched and wide and is usually most prominent in lead II; it is commonly seen in association with mitral valve disease, particularly mitral stenosis (enlarged to show detail).

Table 13.2 Left ventricular hypertrophy.

Voltage criteria
Limb leads
- R wave in lead I plus S wave in lead III >25 mm
- R wave in lead aVL >11 mm
- R wave in lead aVF >20 mm
- S wave in lead aVR >14 mm

Precordial leads
- R wave in leads V4, V5, or V6 > 26 mm
- R wave in leads V5 or 6 plus S wave in lead V1 >35 mm
- Largest R wave plus largest S wave in precordial leads >45 mm

Non-voltage criteria
- Delayed ventricular activation time ≥0.05 s in leads V5 or V6 >0.05 s
- ST segment depression and T wave inversion in the left precordial leads

The specificity of these criteria is age and sex dependent

suggested for the diagnosis of left ventricular hypertrophy, but none is universally accepted. Scoring systems based on these criteria have been developed, and although they are highly specific diagnostic tools, poor sensitivity limits their use.

Electrocardiographic findings

The electrocardiographic features of left ventricular hypertrophy are classified as either voltage criteria or non-voltage criteria.

The electrocardiographic diagnosis of left ventricular hypertrophy is difficult in individuals aged under 40. Voltage criteria lack specificity in this group because young people often have high amplitude QRS complexes in the absence of left ventricular disease. Even when high amplitude QRS complexes are seen in association with non-voltage criteria—such as ST segment and T wave changes—a diagnosis cannot be made with confidence. Typical repolarisation changes seen in left ventricular hypertrophy are ST segment depression and T wave inversion. This "strain" pattern

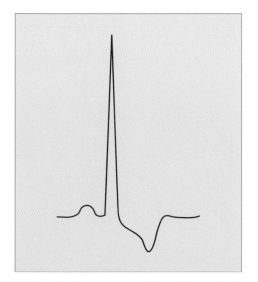

Figure 13.3 Left ventricular hypertrophy with strain (note dominant R wave and repolarisation abnormality).

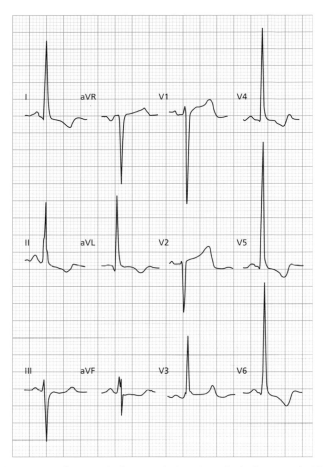

Figure 13.4 Left ventricular hypertrophy in patient who had presented with chest pain and was given thrombolytic therapy inappropriately because of the ST segment changes in V1 and V2.

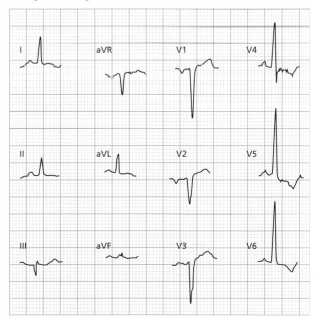

Figure 13.5 Left ventricular hypertrophy without voltage criteria—in a man who presented with heart failure secondary to severe aortic stenosis (gradient 125 mm Hg). The ST segment changes are typical for left ventricular hypertrophy and there is evidence of left atrial enlargement. If the scoring system is used, these findings suggest left ventricular hypertrophy even though none of the R or S waves meets voltage criteria.

is seen in the left precordial leads and is associated with reciprocal ST segment elevation in the right precordial leads.

The presence of these ST segment changes can cause diagnostic difficulty in patients complaining of ischaemic-type chest pain; failure to recognise the features of left ventricular hypertrophy can lead to the inappropriate administration of thrombolytic therapy.

Furthermore, in patients known to have left ventricular hypertrophy it can be difficult to diagnose confidently acute ischaemia on the basis of ST segment changes in the left precordial leads. It is an advantage to have old electrocadiograms for comparison. Other non-voltage criteria are common in left ventricular hypertrophy. Left atrial hypertrophy or prolonged atrial depolarisation and left axis deviation are often present; and poor R wave progression is commonly seen.

The electrocardiogram is abnormal in almost 50% of patients with hypertension, with minimal changes in 20% and obvious features of left ventricular hypertrophy in 30%. There is a linear correlation between the electrocardiographic changes and the severity and duration of the hypertension. High amplitude QRS complexes are seen first, followed by the development of non-voltage criteria.

The specificity of the electrocardiographic diagnosis of left ventricular hypertrophy is improved if a scoring system is used.

Valvular problems

A normal electrocardiogram virtually rules out the presence of severe aortic stenosis, except in congenital valve disease, where the trace may remain normal despite a substantial degree of stenosis. Left ventricular hypertrophy is seen in about 75% of patients with severe aortic stenosis. Left atrial enlargement may also be seen in the electrocardiogram. Left axis deviation and left bundle branch block may occur.

The cardiomyopathies

Diseases of the myocardium are classified into three types on the basis of their functional effects: hypertrophic (obstructed), dilated (congestive), or restrictive cardiomyopathy. In cardiomyopathy the myocardium is diffusely affected, and therefore the resulting electrocardiographic abnormalities may be diverse.

Table 13.3 Scoring system for left ventricular hypertrophy (LVH)—suggested if points total ≥ 5.

Electrocardiographic feature	No of points
Amplitude (any of the following)	3
● Largest R or S wave in limb leads ≥ 20 mm	
● S wave in leads V1 or V2 ≥ 30 mm	
● R wave in leads V5 or V6 ≥ 30 mm	
ST-T wave segment changes typical for LVH in the absence of digitalis	3
Left atrial involvement	3
Left axis deviation	2
QRS duration of ≥ 0.09 s	1
Delayed ventricular activation time in leads V5 and V6 of ≥ 0.05 s	1

Table 13.4 Electrocardiographic features of valvular disease.

● The electrocardiographic features of aortic regurgitation include the features of left ventricular hypertrophy, often with the strain pattern
● Mitral stenosis is associated with left atrial abnormality or atrial fibrillation and right ventricular hypertrophy
● Mitral regurgitation is associated with atrial fibrillation, though again the features of left atrial hypertrophy may be seen if the patient is in sinus rhythm. Evidence of left ventricular hypertrophy may be seen

Common features of cardiomyopathy include electrical holes (Q waves), conduction defects (bundle branch block and axis deviation), and arrhythmias

Table 13.5 Main electrocardiographic changes associated with hypertrophic cardiomyopathy.

● Left ventricular hypertrophy
● Left atrial enlargement
● Abnormal inferior and anterior and/or lateral Q waves
● Bizarre QRS complexes masquerading, for example, as pre-excitation and bundle branch block

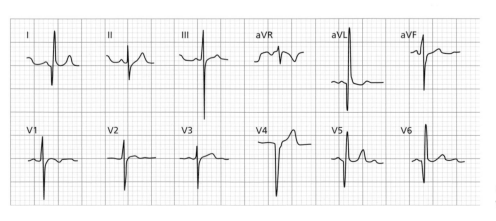

Figure 13.6 Abnormal Q waves in patient with hypertrophic cardiomyopathy.

Hypertrophic cardiomyopathy

This is characterised by marked myocardial thickening predominantly affecting the interventricular septum and/or the apex of the left ventricle. Electrocardiographic evidence of left ventricular hypertrophy is found in 50% of patients. A characteristic abnormality is the presence of abnormal Q waves in the anterolateral or inferior chest leads, which may mimic the appearance of myocardial infarction. As the left ventricle becomes increasingly less compliant, there is increasing resistance to atrial contraction, and signs of left atrial abnormality are commonly seen. Atrial fibrillation and supraventricular tachycardias are common arrhythmias in patients with hypertrophic cardiomyopathy. Ventricular tachycardias may also occur and are a cause of sudden death in these patients.

Dilated cardiomyopathy

Many patients with dilated cardiomyopathy have anatomical left ventricular hypertrophy, though the electrocardiographic signs of left ventricular hypertrophy are seen in only a third of patients. In some patients the signs of left ventricular hypertrophy may be masked as diffuse myocardial fibrosis can reduce the voltage of the QRS complexes. If right ventricular hypertrophy is also present the increased rightward forces of depolarisation may cancel out some of the leftward forces, again masking the signs of left ventricular hypertrophy.

Table 13.6 ECG changes in dilated cardiomyopathy.

- Left bundle branch block
- Left atrial enlargement
- Abnormal Q waves in leads V1 to V4
- Left ventricular hypertrophy
- Arrhythmias—ventricular premature beats, ventricular tachycardia, atrial fibrillation

Adapted from Chou T, Knilans TK. *Electrocardiography in clinical practice*. 4th ed. Philadelphia, PA: Saunders, 1996.

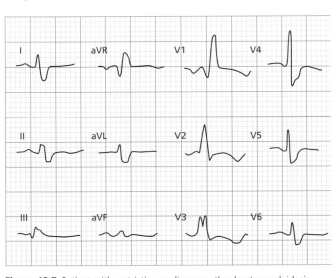

Figure 13.7 Patient with restrictive cardiomyopathy due to amyloidosis (note the low voltage QRS complexes and the right bundle branch block).

Signs of left atrial enlargement are common, and often there is evidence of biatrial enlargement. Abnormal Q waves may be seen, though less commonly than in hypertrophic cardiomyopathy. Abnormal Q waves are most often seen in leads V1 to V4 and may mimic the appearance of a myocardial infarction.

Restrictive cardiomyopathy

Restrictive cardiomyopathy is the least common form of cardiomyopathy and is the end result of several different diseases associated with myocardial infiltration—for example, amyloidosis, sarcoidosis, and haemochromatosis. The most common electrocardiographic abnormality is the presence of low voltage QRS complexes, probably due to myocardial infiltration. Both supraventricular and ventricular arrhythmias are common.

Table 13.7 Electrocardiographic findings in restrictive cardiomyopathy

- Low voltage QRS complexes
- Conduction disturbance
- Arrhythmias—supraventricular, ventricular

Adapted from Chou T, Knilans TK. *Electrocardiography in clinical practice*. 4th ed. Philadelphia, PA: Saunders, 1996.

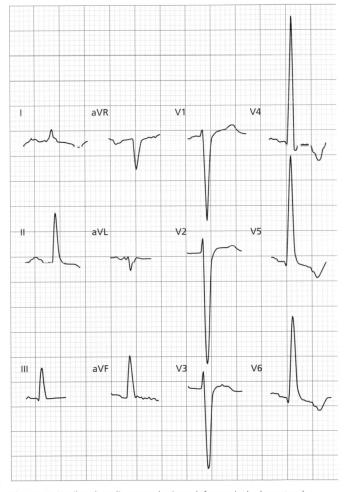

Figure 13.8 Dilated cardiomyopathy (note left ventricular hypertrophy pattern).

CHAPTER 14

Conditions not Primarily Affecting the Heart

Corey Slovis, Richard Jenkins

To function correctly, individual myocardial cells rely on normal concentrations of biochemical parameters such as electrolytes, oxygen, hydrogen, glucose, and thyroid hormones, as well as a normal body temperature. Abnormalities of these and other factors affect the electrical activity of each myocardial cell and thus the surface electrocardiogram. Characteristic electrocardiographic changes may provide useful diagnostic clues to the presence of metabolic abnormalities, the prompt recognition of which can be life saving.

Hyperkalaemia

Increases in total body potassium may have dramatic effects on the electrocardiogram. The most common changes associated with hyperkalaemia are tall, peaked T waves, reduced amplitude and eventually loss of the P wave, and marked widening of the QRS complex.

The earliest changes associated with hyperkalaemia are tall T waves, best seen in leads II, III, and V2 to V4. Tall T waves are usually seen when the potassium concentration rises above 5.5-6.5 mmol/l. However, only about one in five hyperkalaemic patients will have the classic tall, symmetrically narrow and peaked T waves; the rest will merely have large amplitude T waves. Hyperkalaemia should always be suspected when the amplitude of the

It is important to recognise that some electrocardiographic changes are due to conditions other than cardiac disease so that appropriate treatment can be given and unnecessary cardiac investigation avoided

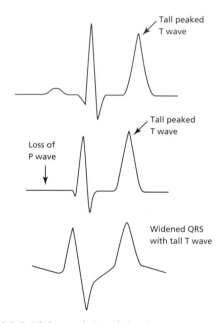

Figure 14.1 Serial changes in hyperkalaemia.

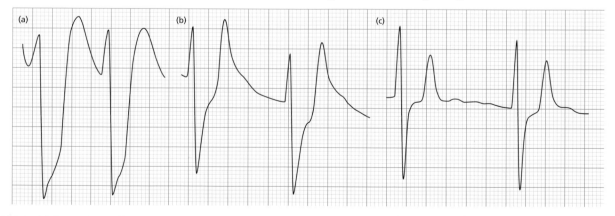

Figure 14.2 Serial changes in patient with renal failure receiving treatment for hyperkalaemia. As potassium concentration drops, the electrocardiogram changes: 9.3 mmol/l, very broad QRS complexes (a); 7.9 mmol/l, wide QRS complexes with peaked T waves and absent P waves (b); 7.2 mmol/l, QRS complex continues to narrow and T waves diminish in size (c).

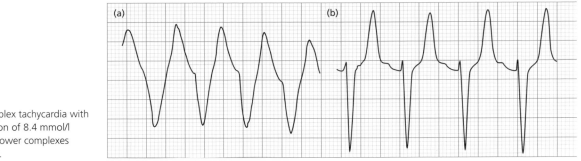

Figure 14.3 Broad complex tachycardia with a potassium concentration of 8.4 mmol/l (a); after treatment, narrower complexes with peaked T waves (b).

T wave is greater than or equal to that of the R wave in more than one lead.

As the potassium concentration rises above 6.5-7.5 mmol/l, changes are seen in the PR interval and the P wave: the P wave widens and flattens and the PR segment lengthens. As the concentration rises, the P waves may disappear.

The QRS complex will begin to widen with a potassium concentration of 7.0-8.0 mmol/l. Unlike right or left bundle branch blocks, the QRS widening in hyperkalaemia affects all portions of the QRS complex and not just the terminal forces. As the QRS complex widens it may begin to merge with the T wave and create a pattern resembling a sine wave—a "preterminal" rhythm. Death resulting from hyperkalaemia may be due to asystole, ventricular fibrillation, or a wide pulseless idioventricular rhythm. Hyperkalaemia induced asystole is more likely to be seen in patients who have had chronic, rather than acute, hyperkalaemia.

Hypokalaemia

Hypokalaemia may produce several electrocardiographic changes, especially when there is total body depletion of both potassium and magnesium. The commonest changes are decreased T wave amplitude, ST segment depression, and presence of a U wave. Other findings, particularly in the presence of coexistent hypomagnesaemia, include a prolonged QT interval, ventricular extrasystoles, and malignant ventricular arrhythmias such as ventricular tachycardia, torsades de pointes, and ventricular fibrillation. Electrocardiographic changes are not common with mild to moderate hypokalaemia, and it is only when serum concentrations are below 2.7 mmol/l that changes reliably appear.

A prominent U wave in association with a small T wave are considered to be the classic electrocardiographic findings of hypokalaemia. Many authors list a prolonged QT interval as a common finding in hypokalaemia. However, most cases of a presumed prolongation of the QT interval are really QU intervals. Most hypokalaemic patients with true prolongation of the QT interval have coexisting hypomagnesaemia and are at risk of ventricular arrhythmias, including torsades de pointes.

Patients with a potassium concentration below 2.5-3.0 mmol/l often develop ventricular extrasystoles. Hypokalaemia may also be associated with supraventricular arrhythmias, such as paroxysmal atrial tachycardia, multifocal atrial tachycardia, atrial fibrillation, and atrial flutter.

Table 14.1 Electrocardiographic features of hyperkalaemia.

Serum potassium (mmol/l)	Major change
5.5-6.5	Tall peaked T waves
6.5-7.5	Loss of P waves
7.0-8.0	Widening of QRS complexes
8.0-10	Sine wave, ventricular arrhythmias, asystole

Table 14.2 Electrocardiographic features of hypokalaemia.

- Broad, flat T waves
- ST depression
- QT interval prolongation
- Ventricular arrhythmias (premature ventricular contractions, torsades de pointes, ventricular tachycardia, ventricular fibrillation)

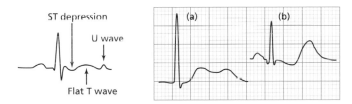

Figure 14.4 Left: Diagram of electrocardiographic changes associated with hypokalaemia. Right: Electrocardiogram showing prominent U wave, potassium concentration 2.5 mmol/l (a) and massive U waves with ST depression and flat T waves, potassium concentration 1.6 mmol/l (b)

Hypothermia

Hypothermia is present when the core temperature is less than 35°C. As body temperature falls below normal, many cardiovascular and electrophysiological changes occur. The earliest change seen in the electrocardiogram is an artefact due to shivering, although some hypothermic patients have relatively normal traces. The ability to shiver diminishes as body temperature falls, and shivering is uncommon below a core temperature of 32°C.

As body temperature falls further, all metabolic and cardiovascular processes slow progressively. Pacemaker (heart rate) and conduction velocity decline, resulting in bradycardia, heart block, and prolongation of the PR, QRS, and QT intervals. At core temperature below 32°C, regular and organised atrial activation disappears and is replaced by varying degrees of slow, irregular, and disorganised activity. If core temperature falls below 28°C, a junctional bradycardia may be seen.

The J wave (Osborn wave) is the most specific electrocardiographic finding in hypothermia. It is considered by many to be pathognomonic for hypothermia, but it may also occasionally be seen in hypercalcaemia and in central nervous system disorders, including massive head injury and subarachnoid haemorrhage.

The J wave may even be a drug effect or, rarely, a normal variant. The J wave is most commonly characterised by a "dome" or "hump" elevation in the terminal portion of the QRS deflection and is best seen in the left chest leads. The size of the J wave often correlates with the severity of hypothermia (< 30°C) but the exact aetiology is not known.

Thyrotoxicosis

The cardiovascular system is very sensitive to increased levels of circulating thyroid hormones. Increases in cardiac output and heart rate are early features in thyrotoxicosis. The most common electrocardiographic changes seen in thyrotoxicosis are sinus tachycardia, an increased electrical amplitude of all deflections, and atrial fibrillation.

About 50% of thyrotoxic patients have a resting pulse rate above 100 beats/min. Atrial tachyarrhythmias are common as the atria are very sensitive to the effects of triiodothyronine. Patients with thyroid storm may develop paroxysmal supraventricular tachycardia with rates exceeding 200 beats/min. Elderly patients may develop ischaemic ST and T wave changes because of their tachycardias. Increased voltage is a common but non-specific electrocardiographic finding in hyperthyroidism, and is more commonly seen in younger patients.

Atrial fibrillation is the most common sustained arrhythmia in thyrotoxicosis, occurring in about 20% of all cases. It is most common in elderly patients, men, those with a particularly high concentration of thyroid hormone, and patients with left atrial enlargement or other intrinsic heart disease. Treatment of atrial fibrillation in thyrotoxicosis is difficult as the rhythm may be refractory to cardioversion. However, most cases revert spontaneously to sinus rhythm when euthyroid. Multifocal atrial tachycardia and atrial flutter with 2:1 conduction, and even 1:1 conduction, may also be seen.

Patients with thyrotoxicosis may have other electrocardiographic findings. Non-specific ST and T wave changes are relatively common. Ventricular arrhythmias may be seen, though much less frequently than atrial arrhythmias. Thyrotoxic patients have two or three times the normal number of premature ventricular contractions.

Hypothyroidism

Hypothyroidism causes slowing of the metabolic rate and affects almost all bodily functions, including heart rate and contractility. It causes similar slowing of electrical conduction throughout the heart.

The most common electrocardiographic changes associated with hypothyroidism are sinus bradycardia, a prolonged QT interval, and inverted or flat T waves. Most hypothyroid patients will have a low to normal heart rate (about 50-70 beats/min). Patients with severe hypothyroidism and those with pre-existing heart disease may also develop increasing degrees of heart block or

Table 14.3 Electrocardiographic features of hypothermia.

- Tremor artefact from shivering
- Atrial fibrillation with slow ventricular rate
- J waves (Osborn waves)
- Bradycardias, especially junctional
- Prolongation of PR, QRS, and QT intervals
- Premature ventricular beats, ventricular tachycardia, or ventricular fibrillation
- Asystole

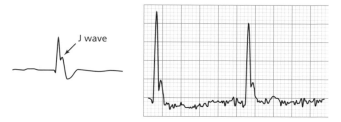

Figure 14.5 Sinus bradycardia, with a J wave, in a patient with hypothermia—core temperature 29°C (note the shivering artefact).

> Ventricular arrhythmias are the most common mechanism of death in hypothermia. They seem to be more common during rewarming as the body temperature rises through the 28°–32°C range

Table 14.4 Electrocardiographic features of thyrotoxicosis.

Most common findings
- Sinus tachycardia
- Increased QRS voltages
- Atrial fibrillation

Other findings
- Supraventricular arrhythmias (premature atrial beats, paroxysmal supraventricular tachycardia, multifocal atrial tachycardia, atrial flutter)
- Non-specific ST and T wave changes
- Ventricular extrasystoles

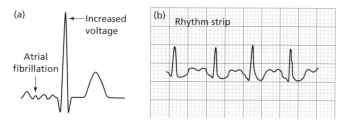
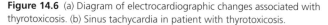

Figure 14.6 (a) Diagram of electrocardiographic changes associated with thyrotoxicosis. (b) Sinus tachycardia in patient with thyrotoxicosis.

bundle branch block (especially right bundle branch block). Conduction abnormalities due to hypothyroidism resolve with thyroid hormone therapy.

Depolarisation, like all phases of the action potential, is slowed in hypothyroidism, and this results in a prolonged QT interval. Torsades de pointes ventricular tachycardia has been reported in hypothyroid patients and is related to prolongation of the QT interval, hypothyroidism induced electrolyte abnormalities, hypothermia, or hypoventilation.

Hypothyroid patients are very sensitive to the effects of digitalis and are predisposed to all the arrhythmias associated with digitalis intoxication.

Uncommonly, patients may develop large pericardial effusions, which give rise to electrical alternans (beat to beat variation in QRS voltages). Myxoedema coma should always be suspected in patients with altered mental states who have bradycardia and low voltage QRS complexes (< 1 mV) in all leads.

Other non-cardiac conditions

Hypercalcaemia is associated with shortening of the QT interval. At high calcium concentrations the duration of the T wave increases and the QT interval may then become normal. Digoxin may be harmful in hypercalcaemic patients and may result in tachyarrhythmias or bradyarrhythmias. Similarly, intravenous calcium may be dangerous in a patient who has received digitalis. The QT prolongation seen in hypocalcaemia is primarily due to ST prolongation but is not thought to be clinically by important.

Hypoglycaemia is a common medical emergency, although it is not often recognised as having electrocardiographic sequelae. The electrocardiographic features include flattening of the T wave and QT prolongation.

Acute electrocardiographic changes commonly accompany severe subarachnoid haemorrhage. Typically these are ST depression or elevation and T wave inversion, although other changes, such as a prolonged QT interval, can also be seen.

Table 14.5 Electrocardiographic features of hypothyroidism.

Most common
- Sinus bradycardia
- Prolonged QT interval
- Flat or inverted T waves

Less common
- Heart block
- Low QRS voltages
- Intraventricular conduction defects
- Ventricular extrasystoles

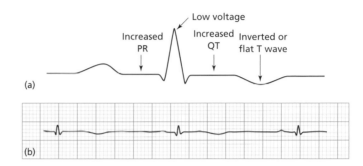

Figure 14.7 (a) Diagram of electrocardiographic changes associated with hypothyroidism. (b) Bradycardia (note small QRS complexes and inverted T waves) in patient with hypothyroidism.

> **Non-specific T wave abnormalities are very common in hypothyroid patients. The T wave may be flattened or inverted in several leads. Unlike with most other causes of T wave abnormalities in hypothyroidism, associated ST changes are rarely seen**

Finally, artefacts due to shivering or tremor can obscure electrocardiographic changes or simulate arrhythmias.

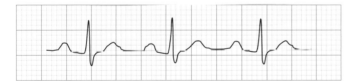

Figure 14.8 Short QT interval in patient with hypercalcaemia (calcium concentration 4 mmol/l).

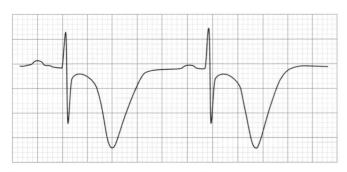

Figure 14.9 Massive T wave inversion and QT prolongation associated with subarachnoid haemorrhage.

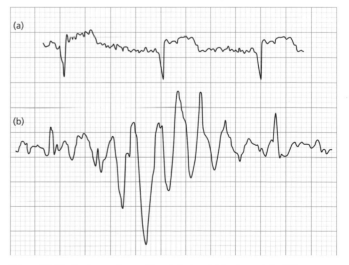

Figure 14.10 Electrocardiographic artefacts—"shivering artefact" in patient with anterior myocardial infarction (a) and electrical interference simulating tachycardia (b).

CHAPTER 15

Paediatric Electrocardiography

Steve Goodacre, Karen McLeod

General clinicians and junior paediatricians may have little experience of interpreting paediatric electrocardiograms. Although the basic principles of cardiac conduction and depolarisation are the same as for adults, age related changes in the anatomy and physiology of infants and children produce normal ranges for electrocardiographic features that differ from adults and vary with age. Awareness of these differences is the key to correct interpretation of paediatric electrocardiograms.

Recording the electrocardiogram

To obtain a satisfactory recording in young children requires patience, and the parents may be helpful in providing a source of distraction. Limb electrodes may be placed in a more proximal position to reduce movement artefacts. Standard adult electrode positions are used but with the addition of either lead V3R or lead V4R to detect right ventricular or atrial hypertrophy. Standard paper speed (25 mm/s) and deflection (10 mm/mV) are used, although occasionally large QRS complexes may require the gain to be halved.

Table 15.1 Successful use of paediatric electrocardiography.

- Be aware of age related differences in the indications for performing electrocardiography, the normal ranges for electrocardiographic variables, and the typical abnormalities in infants and children
- Genuine abnormality is unusual; if abnormality is suspected, seek a specialist opinion

Table 15.2 Indications for paediatric electrocardiography.

• Syncope or seizure	• Electrolyte disturbance
• Exertional symptoms	• Kawasaki disease
• Drug ingestion	• Rheumatic fever
• Tachyarrhythmia	• Myocarditis
• Bradyarrhythmia	• Myocardial contusion
• Cyanotic episodes	• Pericarditis
• Heart failure	• Post cardiac surgery
• Hypothermia	• Congenital heart defects

Table 15.3 Paediatric electrocardiographic findings that may be normal.

- Heart rate > 100 beats/min
- QRS axis > 90°
- Right precordial T wave inversion
- Dominant right precordial R waves
- Short PR and QT intervals
- Short P wave and short duration of QRS complexes
- Inferior and lateral Q waves

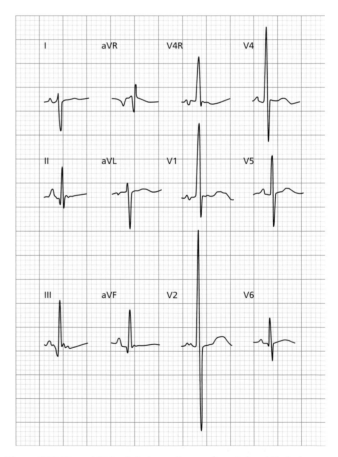

Figure 15.1 Normal 12 lead electrocardiogram from 3 day old baby boy showing right axis deviation, dominant R wave in leads V4R and V1, and still predominantly upright T wave in V1. Persistence of upright T waves in right precordial leads beyond first week of life is sign of right ventricular hypertrophy.

Indications for electrocardiography

Chest pain in children is rarely cardiac in origin and is often associated with tenderness in the chest wall. Electrocardiography is not usually helpful in making a diagnosis, although a normal trace can be very reassuring to the family. Typical indications for paediatric electrocardiography include syncope, exertional symptoms, tachyarrhythmias, bradyarrhythmias, and drug ingestion. Use of electrocardiography to evaluate congenital heart defects is a specialist interest and will not be discussed here.

Age related changes in normal electrocardiograms

Features that would be diagnosed as abnormal in an adult's electrocardiogram may be normal, age related changes in a paediatric trace. The explanation for why this is so lies in how the heart develops during infancy and childhood.

At birth the right ventricle is larger than the left. Changes in systemic vascular resistance result in the left ventricle increasing in size until it is larger than the right ventricle by age 1 month. By age 6 months, the ratio of the right ventricle to the left ventricle is similar to that of an adult. Right axis deviation, large precordial R waves, and upright T waves are therefore normal in the neonate. The T wave in lead V1 inverts by 7 days and typically remains inverted until at least age 7 years. Upright T waves in the right precordial leads (V1 to V3) between ages 7 days and 7 years are a potentially important abnormality and usually indicate right ventricular hypertrophy.

The QRS complex also reflects these changes. At birth, the mean QRS axis lies between + 60° and + 160°, R waves are prominent in the right precordium, and S waves are prominent in the left precordium. By age 1 year, the axis changes gradually to lie between + 10° and + 100°.

The resting heart rate decreases from about 140 beats/min at birth to 120 beats/min at age 1 year, 100 at 5 years, and adult values by 10 years. The PR interval decreases from birth to age 1 year and then gradually increases throughout childhood. The P wave duration and the QRS duration also increase with age. The QT interval depends on heart rate and age, increasing with age while decreasing with heart rate. Q waves are normally seen in the inferior or lateral leads but signify disease if present in other leads.

Abnormal paediatric electrocardiograms

Diagnosis of abnormality on a paediatric electrocardiogram will require knowledge of normal age related values, particularly for criteria relating to right or left ventricular hypertrophy.

P wave amplitude varies little with age and is best evaluated from lead II, V1, or V4R. Wide P waves indicate left atrial hypertrophy, and P waves taller than 2.5 mm in lead II indicate right atrial hypertrophy. P waves showing an abnormal pattern, such as inversion in leads II or aVF, indicate atrial activation from a site other than the sinoatrial node.

Prolongation of the QRS complex may be due to bundle branch block, ventricular hypertrophy, metabolic disturbances, or drugs.

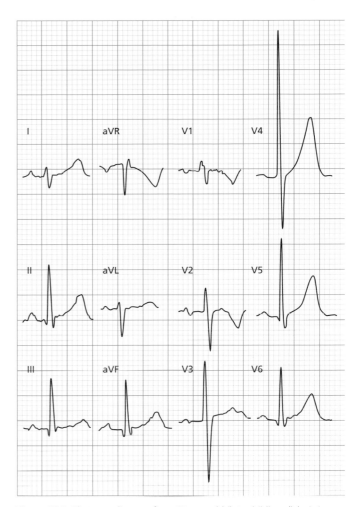

Figure 15.2 Electrocardiogram from 12 year old (late childhood) (axis is now within normal "adult" range and R wave is no longer dominant in right precordial leads).

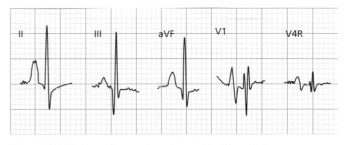

Figure 15.3 Electrocardiogram from 3 year old with restrictive cardiomyopathy and severe right and left atrial enlargement. Tall (>2.5 mm), wide P waves are clearly seen in lead II, and P wave in V1 is markedly biphasic.

Diagnosis of ventricular hypertrophy by "voltage criteria" will depend on age adjusted values for R wave and S wave amplitudes. However, several electrocardiographic features may be useful in making a diagnosis. A qR complex or an rSR′ pattern in lead V1, upright T waves in the right precordial leads between ages 7 days and 7 years, marked right axis deviation (particularly associated with right atrial enlargement), and complete reversal of the adult

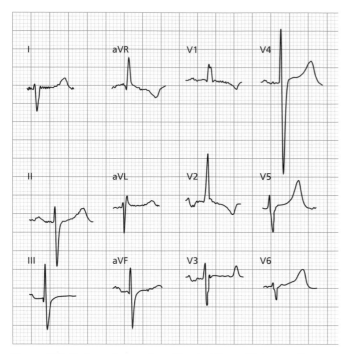

Figure 15.4 Electrocardiogram from 13 year old boy with transposition of great arteries and previous Mustard's procedure. The right ventricle is the systemic ventricle and the trace shows right ventricular hypertrophy with marked right axis deviation and a dominant R wave in the right precordial leads.

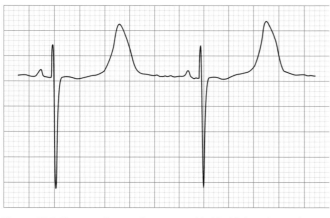

Figure 15.5 Electrocardiogram from 3 year old girl with long QT syndrome.

Table 15.4 Normal values in paediatric electrocardiograms.

Age	PR interval (ms)	QRS duration (ms)	R wave (S wave) amplitude (mm)	
			Lead V1	Lead V6
Birth	80-160	<75	5-26 (1-23)	0-12 (0-10)
6 months	70-150	<75	3-20 (1-17)	6-22 (0-10)
1 year	70-150	<75	2-20 (1-20)	6-23 (0-7)
5 years	80-160	<80	1-16 (2-22)	8-25 (0-5)
10 years	90-170	<85	1-12 (3-25)	9-26 (0-4)

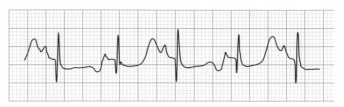

Figure 15.6 Prolongation of QT interval in association with T wave alternans (note alternating upright and inverted T waves).

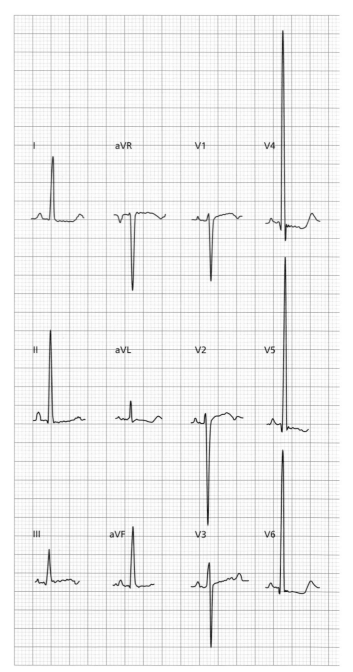

Figure 15.7 Electrocardiogram from 11 year old girl with left ventricular hypertrophy secondary to systemic hypertension. There are tall voltages in the left precordial and limb leads with secondary ST depression and T wave inversion.

precordial pattern of R and S waves will all suggest right ventricular hypertrophy. Left ventricular hypertrophy may be indicated by deep Q waves in the left precordial leads or the typical adult changes of lateral ST depression and T wave inversion.

The QT interval must be corrected for heart rate by dividing its value by the square root of the R-R interval. A corrected QT interval exceeding 0.45 s should be considered prolonged, but it should be noted that the QT interval is highly variable in the first three days of life. QT prolongation may be seen in association with hypokalaemia, hypocalcaemia, hypothermia, drug treatment, cerebral injury, and the congenital long QT syndrome. Other features of the long QT syndrome include notching of the T waves, abnormal U waves, relative bradycardia for age, and T wave alternans. These children may be at risk of ventricular arrhythmia and sudden cardiac death.

Q waves are normally present in leads II, III, aVF, V5, and V6. Q waves in other leads are rare and associated with disease—for example, an anomalous left coronary artery, or myocardial infarction secondary to Kawasaki syndrome.

ST segment elevation may be a normal finding in teenagers as a result of early repolarisation. It may also be seen in myocardial infarction, myocarditis, or pericarditis.

In addition to the changes seen in ventricular hypertrophy, T waves may be inverted as a result of myocardial disease (inflammation, infarction, or contusion). Flat T waves are seen in association with hypothyroidism. Abnormally tall T waves occur with hyperkalaemia.

Abnormalities of rate and rhythm

The wide variation in children's heart rate with age and activity may lead to misinterpretation by those more used to adult electrocardiography. Systemic illness must be considered in any child presenting with an abnormal cardiac rate or rhythm. Sinus tachycardia in babies and infants can result in rates of up to 240 beats/min, and hypoxia, sepsis, acidosis, or intracranial lesions may cause bradycardia. Sinus arrhythmia is a common feature in children's electrocardiograms and is often quite marked. Its relation to breathing—slowing on expiration and speeding up on inspiration—allows diagnosis.

The approach to electrocardiographic diagnosis of tachyarrhythmias in children is similar to that used in adults. Most narrow complex tachycardias in children are due to atrioventricular re-entrant tachycardia secondary to an accessory pathway. If the pathway conducts only retrogradely, the electrocardiogram in sinus rhythm will be normal and the pathway is said to be "concealed." If the pathway conducts anterogradely in sinus rhythm, then the trace will show the typical features of the Wolff-Parkinson-White syndrome. AV nodal re-entrant tachycardia is rare in infants but may be seen in later childhood and adolescence.

Atrial flutter and fibrillation are rare in childhood and are usually associated with underlying structural heart disease or previous cardiac surgery. Atrial flutter can present as an uncommon arrhythmia in neonates with apparently otherwise normal hearts.

Table 15.5 Extrasystoles.

- Atrial extrasystoles are very common and rarely associated with disease
- Ventricular extrasystoles are also common and, in the context of the structurally normal heart, are almost always benign
- Typically, atrial and ventricular extrasystoles are abolished by exercise

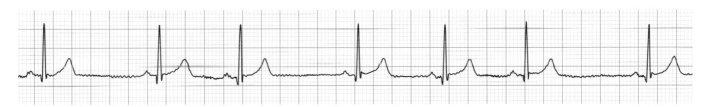

Figure 15.8 Electrocardiogram from 9 year old boy showing marked sinus arrhythmia, a common finding in paediatric traces.

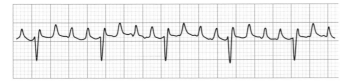

Figure 15.9 Electrocardiogram showing atrial "flutter" in 14 year old girl with congenital heart disease and previous atrial surgery (in neonates with atrial flutter, 1:1 atrioventricular conduction is more common, which may make P waves and diagnosis less evident).

Aids for diagnosing tachycardias, such as atrioventricular dissociation and capture and fusion beats, are less common in children than in adults

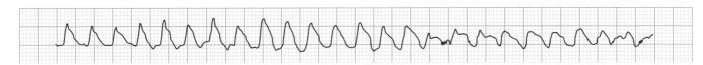

Figure 15.10 Polymorphic ventricular tachycardia in 5 year old girl.

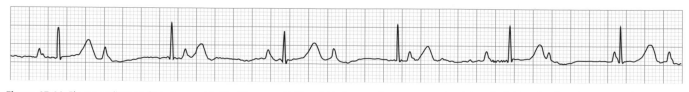

Figure 15.11 Electrocardiogram from 6 year old girl with congenital heart block secondary to maternal antiphospholipid antibodies; there is complete atrioventricular dissociation, and the ventricular escape rate is about 50 beats/min.

Although all forms of ventricular tachycardia are rare, broad complex tachycardia should be considered to be ventricular tachycardia until proved otherwise. Bundle branch block (usually right bundle) often occurs after cardiac surgery, and a previous electrocardiogram can be helpful. Monomorphic ventricular tachycardia may occur secondary to surgery for congenital heart disease. Polymorphic ventricular tachycardia, or torsades de pointes, is associated with the long QT syndrome.

Classification of atrioventricular block into first, second, and third degree follows the same principles as for adults, although a diagnosis of first degree heart block should take into account the variation of the PR interval with age. First degree heart block and the Wenckebach phenomenon may be a normal finding in otherwise healthy children. First or second degree block, however, can occur with rheumatic carditis, diphtheria, digoxin overdose, and congenital heart defects.

Table 15.6 Complete atrioventricular block.

- Complete atrioventricular block may be congenital or secondary to surgery
- An association exists between congenital complete atrioventricular block and maternal anti-La and anti-Ro antibodies, which are believed to cross the placenta and damage conduction tissue

CHAPTER 16

Cardiac Arrest Rhythms

Robert French, Daniel DeBehnke, Stephen Hawes

Successful resuscitation from cardiac arrest depends on prompt recognition and appropriate treatment of the arrest rhythm. Arrhythmias are frequent immediately before and after arrest; some are particularly serious because they may precipitate cardiac arrest—for example, ventricular tachycardia frequently deteriorates into fibrillation. Early recognition of such arrhythmias is therefore vital, necessitating cardiac monitoring of vulnerable patients.

The cardiac arrest rhythms are ventricular fibrillation, pulseless ventricular tachycardia, pulseless electrical activity (also termed electromechanical dissociation), and asystole.

In pulseless ventricular tachycardia and electromechanical dissociation, organised electrical activity is present but fails to produce a detectable cardiac output. In ventricular fibrillation the electrical activity is disorganised, and in asystole it is absent altogether.

Ventricular fibrillation is usually a primary cardiac event, and with early direct current cardioversion the prognosis is relatively good. By contrast, asystole and electromechanical dissociation have a poor prognosis, with survival dependent on the presence of a treatable underlying condition.

Ventricular fibrillation

Mechanisms

Ventricular fibrillation probably begins in a localised area from which waves of activation spread in all directions.

The individual myocardial cells contract in an uncoordinated, rapid fashion. Fibrillation seems to be maintained by the continuous re-entry of waves of activation. Activation is initially rapid but slows as the myocardium becomes increasingly ischaemic.

Electrocardiographic features

The chaotic myocardial activity is reflected in the electrocardiogram, with rapid irregular deflections of varying amplitude and

Table 16.1 Cardiac arrest rhythms.

- Ventricular fibrillation
- Pulseless ventricular tachycardia
- Pulseless electrical activity (electromechanical dissociation)
- Asystole

Ventricular fibrillation is the commonest arrhythmia that causes sudden death out of hospital

Table 16.2 Causes of ventricular fibrillation.

- Myocardial ischaemia/infarction
- Cardiomyopathy
- Acidosis
- Electrocution
- Drugs (for example—quinidine, digoxin, tricyclic antidepressants)
- Electrolyte disturbance (for example—hypokalaemia)

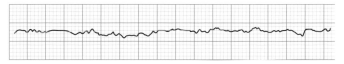

Figure 16.1 Fine ventricular fibrillation.

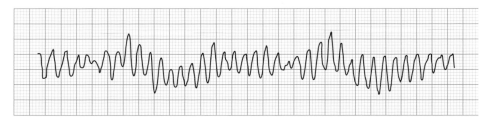

Figure 16.2 Coarse ventricular fibrillation.

morphology and no discernible QRS complexes. The deflection rate varies between 150 and 500 beats/min. Although the atria may continue to beat, no P waves are usually discernible. Ventricular fibrillation may be termed "coarse" or "fine" depending on the amplitude of the deflections.

Initially, ventricular fibrillation tends to be high amplitude (coarse) but later degenerates to fine ventricular fibrillation.

Potential pitfalls in diagnosis

When the amplitude of the deflections is extremely low, fine ventricular fibrillation can be mistaken for asystole. To avoid this mistake, check the "gain" (wave form amplitude) on the electrocardiogram machine in case it has been set at an inappropriately low level. In addition, check the trace from two leads perpendicular to one another (for example, leads II and aVL) because occasionally a predominant ventricular fibrillation wave form vector may occur perpendicular to the sensing electrode and appear as an almost flat line.

"Persistent movement artefact," such as that which occurs in a patient who is fitting, can simulate ventricular fibrillation

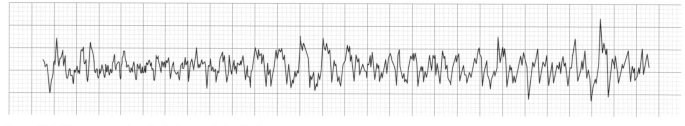

Figure 16.3 Movement artefact simulating ventricular fibrillation.

Electrocardiographic predictors

Acute myocardial ischaemia or infarction, especially anterior infarction, is commonly associated with ventricular arrhythmias. Ventricular fibrillation is often preceded by episodes of sustained or non-sustained ventricular tachycardia. Frequent premature ventricular beats may herald the onset of ventricular fibrillation, especially if they occur when the myocardium is only partially repolarised (the "R on T" phenomenon), though in the ischaemic myocardium the ventricles are probably vulnerable during all phases of the cardiac cycle. T wave alternans, a regular beat to beat change in T wave amplitude, is also thought to predict ventricular fibrillation.

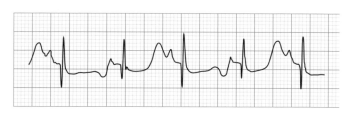

Figure 16.4 T wave alternans.

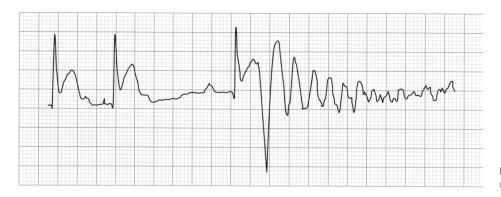

Figure 16.5 "R on T" phenomenon giving rise to ventricular fibrillation.

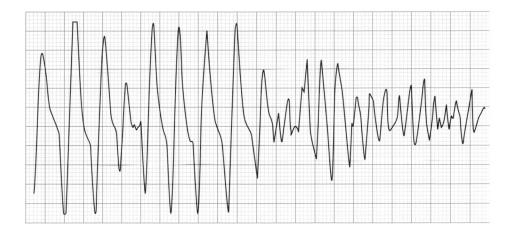

Figure 16.6 Polymorphic ventricular tachycardia deteriorating into ventricular fibrillation.

Pulseless ventricular tachycardia

Ventricular tachycardias are the result of increased myocardial automaticity or are secondary to a re-entry phenomenon. They can result from direct myocardial damage secondary to ischaemia, cardiomyopathy, or myocarditis or be caused by drugs—for example, class 1 antiarrhythmics such as flecainide and disopyramide. Pulseless ventricular tachycardia is managed in the same way as ventricular fibrillation, early defibrillation being the mainstay of treatment.

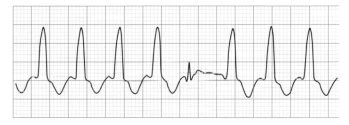

Figure 16.7 Capture beat in ventricular tachycardia.

Electrocardiographic features

In a patient who is in the middle of a cardiac arrest 12 lead electrocardiography is impractical; use a cardiac monitor to determine the rhythm, and any broad complex tachycardia should be assumed to be ventricular in origin.

In ventricular tachycardia there is a broad complex, regular tachycardia with a rate of at least 120 beats/min. The diagnosis is confirmed if there is direct or indirect evidence of atrioventricular dissociation, such as capture beat, fusion beat, or independent P wave activity.

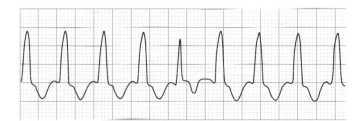

Figure 16.8 Fusion beat in ventricular tachycardia.

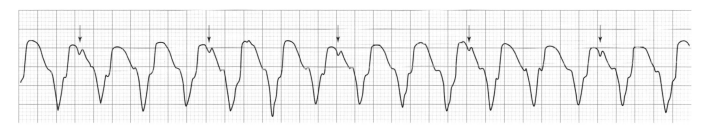

Figure 16.9 Ventricular tachycardia with evidence of atrioventricular dissociation.

Pulseless electrical activity

In pulseless electrical activity the heart continues to work electrically but fails to provide a cardiac output sufficient to produce a palpable pulse.

Electrocardiographic features of pulseless electrical activity

The appearance of the electrocardiogram varies, but several common patterns exist. There may be a normal sinus rhythm or sinus

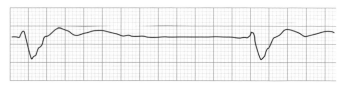

Figure 16.10 Broad and slow rhythm in association with pulseless electrical activity.

tachycardia, with discernible P waves and QRS complexes. Sometimes there is a bradycardia, with or without P waves, and often with wide QRS complexes.

Clinical correlates

Successful treatment of pulseless electrical activity depends on whether it is a primary cardiac event or is secondary to a potentially reversible disorder.

Table 16.3 Potentially reversible causes of pulseless electrical activity.

- Hypovolaemia
- Cardiac tamponade
- Tension pneumothorax
- Massive pulmonary embolism
- Hyperkalaemia, hypokalaemia, and metabolic disorders
- Hypothermia
- Toxic disturbances—for example, overdoses of β blockers, tricyclic antidepressants, or calcium channel blockers

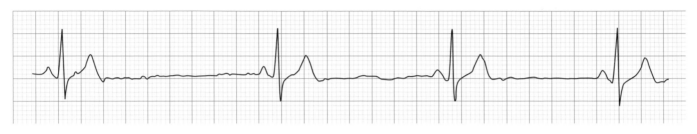

Figure 16.11 Narrow complex rhythm associated with pulseless electrical activity.

Asystole

Mechanisms

Asystole implies the absence of any cardiac electrical activity. It results from a failure of impulse formation in the pacemaker tissue or from a failure of propagation to the ventricles. Ventricular and atrial asystole usually coexist. Asystole may be structurally mediated (for example, in acute myocardial infarction), neurally mediated (for example, in aortic stenosis), or secondary to antiarrhythmic drugs.

Electocardiographic features of asystole

In asystole the electrocardiogram shows an almost flat line. Slight undulations are present because of baseline drift. There are several potential pitfalls in the diagnosis of asystole. A completely flat trace indicates that a monitoring lead has become disconnected, so check that the leads are correctly attached to the patient and the monitor. Check the electrocardiogram gain in case it has been set at an inappropriately low level. To eliminate the possibility of mistaking fine ventricular fibrillation for asystole, check the trace from two perpendicular leads.

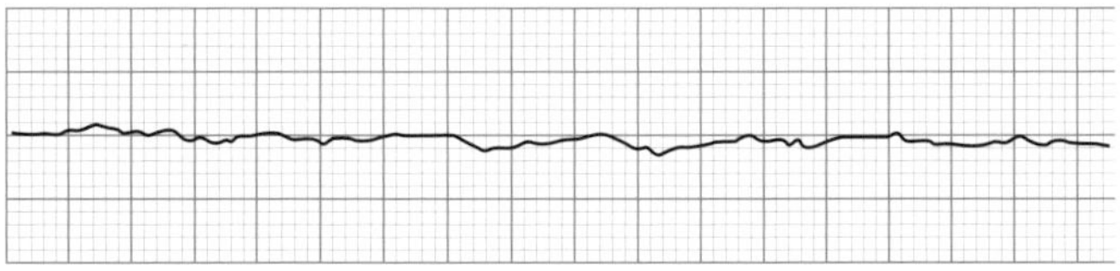

Figure 16.12 Asystole.

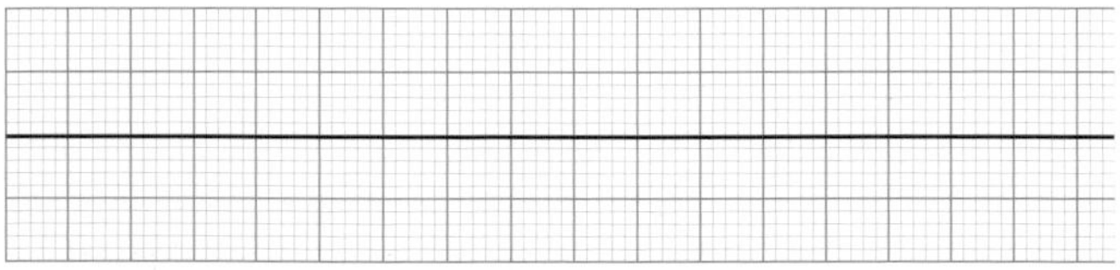

Clinical correlates

Asystole has the worst prognosis of all the arrest rhythms. If ventricular fibrillation cannot be excluded confidently, make an attempt at defibrillation.

Figure 16.13 Flat line artefact simulating asystole.

Ventricular standstill

Atrial activity may continue for a short time after ventricular activity has stopped and the electrocardiogram shows a flat line interrupted by only P waves. Conduction abnormalities that can herald ventricular standstill include trifascicular block and the occurrence of alternating left and right bundle branch block.

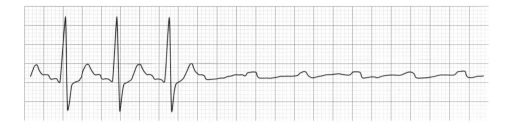

Figure 16.14 Ventricular standstill.

Bradycardias and conduction blocks

The term bradycardia refers to rates of < 60 beats/min, but a relative bradycardia exists when the rate is too slow for the haemodynamic state of the patient. Some bradycardias may progress to asystole, and prophylactic transvenous pacing may be needed. These include Mobitz type II block, complete heart block with a wide QRS complex, symptomatic pauses lasting three seconds or more, and where there is a history of asystole.

At low heart rates, escape beats may arise from subsidiary pacemaker tissue in the atrioventricular junction or ventricular myocardium. A junctional escape rhythm usually has a rate of 40-60 beats/min; the QRS morphology is normal, but inverted P waves may be apparent. Ventricular escape rhythms are usually slower (15-40 beats/min), with broad QRS complexes and no P waves.

Table 16.4 "Peri-arrest" rhythms.

- Arrhythmias are common immediately before and after arrest, and cardiac monitoring of patients at high risk is important
- These "peri-arrest" arrhythmias include bradycardias and conduction blocks, broad complex tachycardias, and narrow complex tachycardias

> Escape rhythms represent a safety net preventing asystole or extreme bradycardia; management should correct the underlying rhythm abnormality

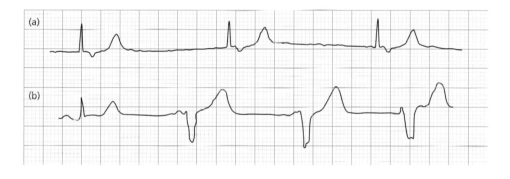

Figure 16.15 (a) Junctional escape rhythm. (b) Ventricular escape rhythm.

Broad complex tachycardias

Management of ventricular tachycardia precipitating cardiac arrest depends on the patient's clinical state. However, some types of ventricular tachycardia warrant special mention.

Polymorphic ventricular tachycardia

In polymorphic ventricular tachycardia, the QRS morphology varies from beat to beat. The rate is usually greater than 200 beats/min. In sinus rhythm the QT interval is normal. If sustained, polymorphic ventricular tachycardia invariably leads to haemodynamic collapse. It often occurs in association with acute myocardial infarction, and frequently deteriorates into ventricular fibrillation.

Torsades de pointes

Torsades de pointes is a type of polymorphic ventricular tachycardia in which the cardiac axis rotates over a sequence of about 5-20 beats, changing from one direction to the opposite direction and back again. In sinus rhythm the QT interval is prolonged, and prominent U waves may be seen.

> Ventricular tachyarrhythmias often precipitate cardiac arrest, and they are common immediately after arrest

> Polymorphic ventricular tachycardia requires immediate direct current cardioversion

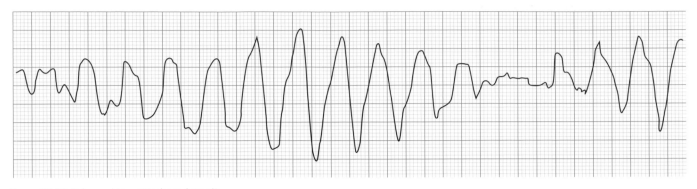

Figure 16.16 Polymorphic ventricular tachycardia.

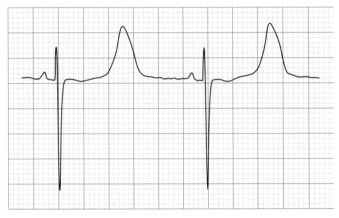

Figure 16.17 Prolonged QT interval.

Torsades de pointes tachycardia is not usually sustained but is recurrent, each bout lasting about 90 s. It may be drug induced, secondary to electrolyte disturbances, or associated with congenital syndromes with prolongation of the QT interval. Its recognition is important because antiarrhythmic drugs have a deleterious effect; management entails reversing the underlying cause. Occasionally torsades de pointes is associated with cardiac arrest or degenerates into ventricular fibrillation; both are managed by direct current cardioversion.

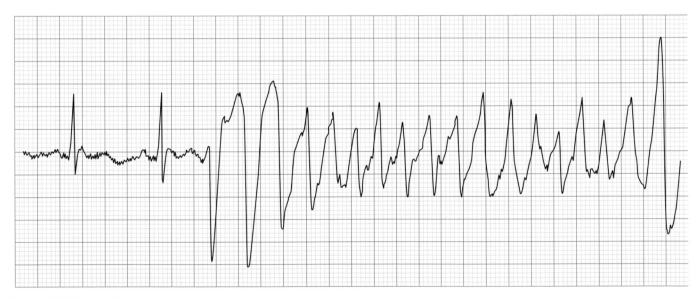

Figure 16.18 Torsades de pointes.

CHAPTER 17

Pacemakers and Electrocardiography

Richard Harper, Francis Morris

Since the placement of the first implantable electronic pacemaker in the 1950s, pacemakers have become increasingly common and complex. The first pacemakers were relatively simple devices consisting of an oscillator, battery, and stimulus generator. They provided single chamber pacing at a single fixed rate irrespective of the underlying rhythm. The second generation of pacemaker had an amplifier and sensing circuit to recognise spontaneous cardiac activity and postpone pacing stimuli until a pause or bradycardia occurred.

Clinical relevance

Pacemakers are implanted primarily for the treatment of symptomatic bradycardia. Modern units have an average life span of about eight years and rarely malfunction.

In clinical practice a basic understanding of electrocardiography in patients with a pacemaker may be helpful in evaluating patients with syncope or near syncope (suggesting that the pacemaker may not be functioning normally).

Troubleshooting potential pacemaker problems is a highly specialised area that needs a skilled technician to evaluate whether the pacemaker is functioning correctly. This field is beyond the scope of this chapter, which will concentrate on basic interpretation of electrocardiograms in the patients who have a pacemaker.

Functions of pacemakers

Pacemakers can pace the ventricle or the atrium, or both sequentially. Atrial or ventricular activity can be sensed, and this sensing may be used to trigger or inhibit pacer activity. Some pacemakers are rate adaptive.

The functions of a pacemaker are indicated by a generic code accepted by the North American Society for Pacing and Electrophysiology and the British Pacing and Electrophysiology Group. It is a five letter code of which only the first four letters are used commonly.[*] The first letter identifies the chamber paced, the second gives the chamber sensed, the third letter indicates the response to sensing, and the fourth identifies rate responsiveness.

AAI pacing

AAI pacing is restricted to those patients with underlying sinus node dysfunction but intact cardiac conduction. This mode will

> **Modern pacemakers can sequentially pace the right atrium or the ventricle, or both, and adapt the discharge frequency of the pacemaker to the patient's physiological needs**

Table 17.1 Indications for a permanent pacemaker system.

- Sick sinus syndrome
- Complete heart block
- Mobitz-type II heart block
- Atrial tachycardia, and heart block
- Asystole
- Carotid sinus hypersensitivity

Table 17.2 Generic pacemaker code.

Chamber paced	Chamber sensed	Response to sensing	Rate modulation*	Anti tachycardia AICDs
O = none	O = none	O = none	O = none	O = none
A = atrium	A = atrium	T = triggered	R = rate responsive	P = pacing
V = ventricle	V = ventricle	I = inhibited		S = shock
D = dual chamber	D = dual chamber	D = dual (T + I)		D = dual (P+S)

*This position may also be used to indicate the degree of programmability by the codes P, M and C.
AICD = Automatic implantable cardioverter defibrillator.

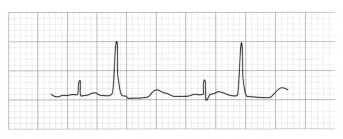

Figure 17.1 Typical electrocardiogram produced by AAI pacing.

sense atrial activity and inhibit pacing if the patient's heart rate remains above the preset target. At lower rates the pacer stimulates the atrium. Like all pacemakers, an AAI pacemaker can be rate adaptive (AAIR).

VVI pacing

VVI pacing is used in patients who do not have useful atrial function, including those with chronic atrial fibrillation or flutter and those with silent atria.

VVI pacing tracks only ventricular activity and paces the ventricle if a QRS complex is not sensed within a predefined interval. VVI pacing may be used as a safety net in patients who are unlikely to need more than occasional pacing.

Dual chamber pacing

Dual chamber pacing has become more common as accumulated evidence shows that sequential dual chamber pacing provides a better quality of life and improved functional capacity for patients. In DDD mode an atrial impulse is generated if the patient's natural atrial activity fails to occur within a preset time period after the last atrial or ventricular event. An atrial event (paced or sensed) begins the atrioventricular interval. If a spontaneous QRS complex does not occur during the programmed atrioventricular interval, a ventricular stimulus is generated. The ventricular stimulus, or sensed QRS complex, initiates a refractory period of the atrial amplifier known as the postventricular atrial refractory period. The combination of the atrioventricular interval and the postventricular atrial refractory period form the total atrial refractory period. The total atrial refractory period is important because it determines the upper rate limit of the pacemaker.

Normal paced rhythm

For implanted pacemakers, the atrial lead is placed in the right atrium and often in the appendage. A beat that is paced has a P wave of near normal appearance. The ventricular lead is placed in the apex of the right ventricle. When the lead is stimulated it produces a wave of depolarisation that spreads through the myocardium, bypassing the normal conduction system. The ventricles depolarise from right to left and from apex to base. This usually produces an electrocardiogram with broad QRS complexes, a left bundle branch block pattern, and left axis deviation. The QT interval is often prolonged and the T waves are broad with a polarity opposite to that of the QRS.

Pacing spikes in the electrocardiogram vary in size and are affected by respiration. Unipolar systems common in the United Kingdom give rise to larger spikes than bipolar systems. Spikes from bipolar systems can be so small that they cannot be seen in the electrocardiogram, especially when single leads are recorded.

Pacemakers are normally programmed to pace at a rate of 70 beats/min (lower rate limit). However, many pacemaker systems are programmed to initiate pacing only when the intrinsic (the patient's own) heart rate drops as low as 50 or 60 beats/min. Therefore, an electrocardiogram with no pacing spikes and with a spontaneous heart rate of 66 beats/min does not necessarily mean the pacemaker has malfunctioned. Heart rates above the lower rate limit will inhibit pacemaker activity, and therefore

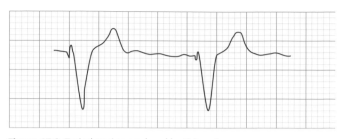

Figure 17.2 Typical tracing produced by VVI pacing.

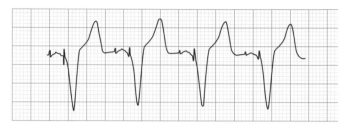

Figure 17.3 Typical tracing produced by DDD pacer.

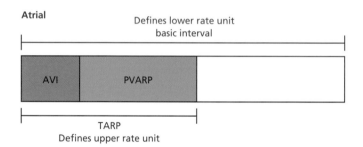
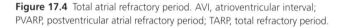

Figure 17.4 Total atrial refractory period. AVI, atrioventricular interval; PVARP, postventricular atrial refractory period; TARP, total refractory period.

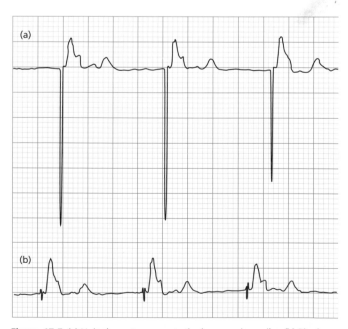

Figure 17.5 (a) Unipolar systems—note the large pacing spike. (b) Bipolar system in the same patient.

electrocardiography will not help in assessing whether the pacemaker is functioning correctly. When this occurs carotid sinus massage can slow the intrinsic rate sufficiently to trigger pacemaker activity.

Alternatively, placing a magnet over the pacemaker will convert the pacer to asynchronous mode so that all sensing is disabled. Ventricular pacers operate in VOO mode, atrial pacers in AOO mode, and dual chamber pacers in DOO mode. If pacing suppresses the native rhythm, a completely paced electrocardiogram at a preset "magnet rate" will result. Many pacemakers have a preset "magnet rate" of 90-100 beats/min. This will usually suppress the native rhythm, allowing the functioning of the pacemaker to be assessed. Removing the magnet will cause the pacemaker to revert to its programmed mode.

Pacemaker failure

Several procedures are needed to assess a patient whose pacemaker may be malfunctioning: cardiac monitoring to assess rhythm disturbances; 12 lead electrocardiography to assess pacer function; and chest x-ray examination to check electrode placement and exclude lead fracture. A patient presenting with pacemaker failure will often have a recurrence of symptomatic bradycardia. If this is captured on a monitor, the diagnosis is confirmed.

Abnormalities of sensing

Undersensing

Undersensing occurs when the pacemaker intermittently or persistently fails to sense the appropriate cardiac chamber, and therefore the timing of the pacemaker stimulus is inappropriate. These mistimed pacemaker spikes may or may not capture the heart, depending on their time of occurrence—for example, spikes occurring soon after spontaneous activity will not capture the relevant chamber because it is still refractory.

Oversensing

Pacemakers may sense electrograms evoked by the pacemaker itself, spontaneous T waves, or electrograms from another chamber,

Table 17.3 Procedures to assess a possible pacemaker malfunction.

- Cardiac monitoring
- 12 lead electrocardiography
- Chest x-ray examination

> Failure to sense may be caused by fibrosis at the tip of the electrode, damage to the electrode or lead, or dislodgment of the lead

> Reprogramming the pacemaker may eliminate the oversensing by adjusting amplifier sensitivity and refractoriness

myopotentials, electromagnetic signals, radio signals, or spikes resulting from lead damage or circuit faults. The sensed signals are misinterpreted as spontaneous electrograms from the appropriate cardiac chamber, and the result is pacemaker inhibition. This can lead to symptomatic bradycardia. The pacemaker system may need to be replaced if there are problems with the circuit, electrodes, or leads.

Failure to pace

Failure to pace is a common reason for pacemaker malfunction and may be caused by failure of the pacemaker to provide output or failure of the pacemaker stimulus to capture. Failure of the pacemaker to provide output should be suspected when the patient's heart rate is below the pacer rate and no pacemaker activity is noted in the electrocardiogram.

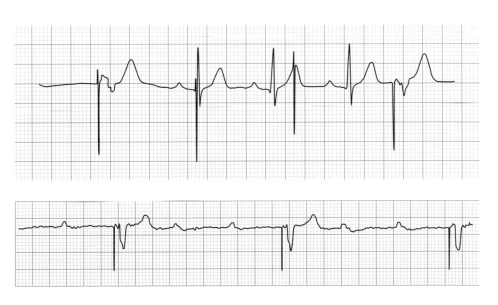

Figure 17.6 Loss of ventricular sensing. The first and the fifth complexes are ventricular paced beats. The second to fourth complexes are the patient's intrinsic rhythm, which have not been sensed, hence the inappropriately timed pacing spike.

Figure 17.7 Loss of atrial pacing because of oversensing preceding T wave. Ventricular pacing set at a low rate.

Failure to capture

Failure to capture should be easy to detect in the electrocardiogram. Appropriately timed pacer spikes will be present, but the spikes fail to provide consistent capture. The commonest cause of loss of capture is dislodgment of the pacing electrode. Failure to capture may also result from lead damage or pacemaker failure (rare).

Table 17.4 Causes of failure to capture.

Failure of pacemaker
- Battery failure
- Circuit abnormality
- Inappropriate programming
- Problem with leads
- Lead dislodgment
- Cardiac perforation
- Lead fracture
- Insulation break
- Increased threshold

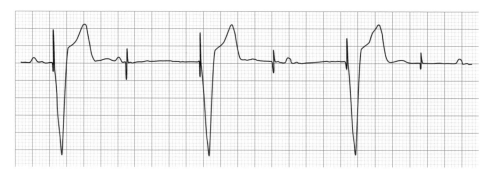

Figure 17.8 VVI pacemaker with intermittent failure to capture. Every second pacemaker beat captures. The rest of the time, pacemaker spikes are seen but not associated with capture.

Pacemaker mediated tachycardias

Pacemaker mediated tachycardias are a result of interactions between native cardiac activity and the pacemaker. In "endless loop tachycardia," a premature ventricular contraction is followed by retrograde atrial conduction. The pacemaker senses the retrograde atrial activity and a ventricular stimulus is generated. If the retrograde conduction persists, a tachycardia ensues. The rate of this tachycardia will not exceed the maximum tracking rate of the pacemaker and is therefore unlikely to result in instability. However, it is often highly symptomatic. Appropriate reprogramming will usually eliminate endless loop tachycardia. Other premature ventricular contractions include rapid ventricular pacing in response to the sensing of atrial tachycardias such as atrial fibrillation.

> The most commonly reported pacemaker mediated tachycardia is "endless loop tachycardia" which occurs in patients with dual chamber pacemakers

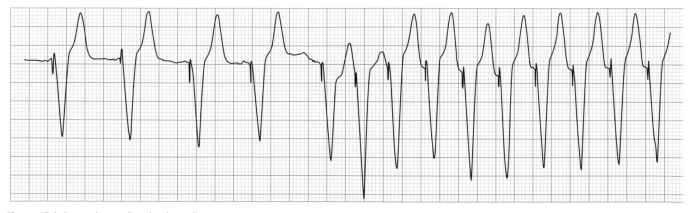

Figure 17.9 Pacemaker mediated tachycardia.

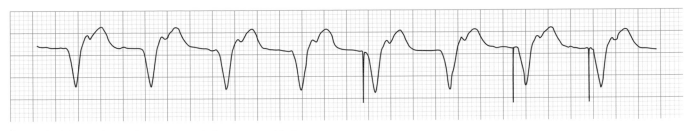

Figure 17.10 Pacemaker syndrome: retrograde P waves are evident.

Pacemaker syndrome

Pacemaker syndrome refers to symptoms related to the use of a pacemaker. When the atria and ventricles contract at the same time the atrial contribution to ventricular filling is lost. It is patients with ventricular pacemakers who are usually affected by pacemaker syndrome. Ventricular pacing leads to retrograde conduction to the atria. The atria contract against closed atrioventricular valves, and this results in pulmonary and systemic venous distension, hypotension, and reduced cardiac output. The diagnosis is largely clinical but may be supported by the presence of retrograde P waves in the electrocardiogram.

Table 17.5 Symptoms of pacemaker syndrome.

- Patients usually present with non-specific symptoms and signs such as dyspnoea, dizziness, fatigue, orthopnoea, and confusion
- Occasionally patients may complain of palpitations or pulsation in the neck or abdomen

CHAPTER 18

Pericarditis, Myocarditis, Drug Effects, and Congenital Heart Disease

Chris A Ghammaghami, Jennifer H Lindsey

Pericarditis, myocarditis, drugs, and some congenital heart lesions all have various effects on the electrocardiogram that can help both in diagnosing a clinical syndrome and monitoring disease progression or resolution.

Pericarditis

The clinical presentation of pericarditis must be differentiated from chest pain related to ischaemic heart disease. Although a careful history and physical examination help to distinguish the two diagnoses, the electrocardiographic changes of pericarditis have at least two characteristic features.

Firstly, in pericarditis the ST segment elevation evolves over time, is "saddle shaped" (concave upwards), widespread, and, with the exception of ST segment depression in lead aVR, is not associated with reciprocal changes.

Secondly, a common though subtle finding in pericarditis is the presence of PR segment depression, which indicates atrial involvement in the inflammatory process. A reduction in QRS voltage and, rarely, electrical alternans of the QRST complex can be seen in patients developing a large pericardial effusion.

Myocarditis

The electrocardiographic findings in myocarditis are usually manifest in two distinct patterns: impairment of conduction, leading to atrioventricular, fascicular, or bundle branch blocks; and widespread ST and T wave changes. Diffuse T wave inversion, which may be associated with ST segment depression, is one of the most common findings.

A resting sinus tachycardia can indicate early myocarditis. Later in the course of the disease, as ventricular function begins to fail, serious arrhythmias are more common. Premature atrial and ventricular contractions can be followed by atrial fibrillation or flutter, and, in late stages, ventricular tachycardia and fibrillation.

Drugs

Each agent in the Vaughan-Williams classification of antiarrhythmic drug actions can cause electrocardiographic changes.

β adrenergic receptor and non-dihydropyridine calcium channel antagonists produce sinus bradycardia and atrioventricular

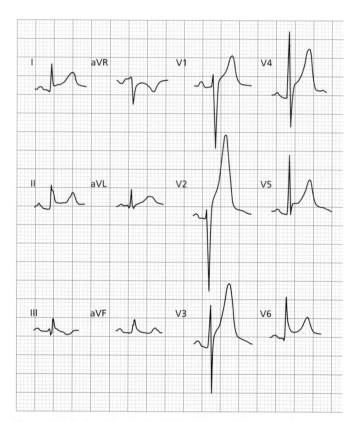

Figure 18.1 Pericarditis: note the ST elevation and PR segment depression.

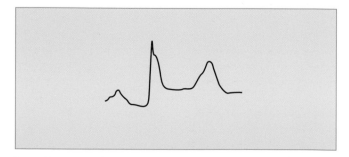

Figure 18.2 Pericarditis: details of the QRS complex in lead II (note the PR segment depression).

block. Generally these drugs are safe and rarely cause severe bradycardia.

Digoxin and quinidine-like agents have narrower therapeutic indices and can cause life threatening ventricular arrhythmias relatively often. Drugs which prolong the action potential duration (class Ia or class III) may cause torsades de pointes. Powerful class I drugs (especially Ia or Ic) may cause QRS widening, bundle branch block, or complete atrioventricular block.

Digoxin

Decades of clinical experience with digitalis compounds show that nearly any arrhythmia can occur as a result of digoxin administration. At therapeutic levels QT duration is shortened, and the PR interval is moderately lengthened because of increased vagal tone. The "digoxin effect" refers to T wave inversion and downsloping ST segment depression. These findings should not be interpreted as toxic effects. Excitatory and inhibitory effects are responsible for the pro-arrhythmic character of digoxin. A rhythm that is considered by some as nearly pathognomonic for digoxin intoxication, paroxysmal atrial tachycardia with variable atrioventricular nodal conduction ("PAT with block"), shows both types of effects.

Table 18.1 Vaughan-Williams classification.

Class I: Fast sodium channel blockers
- 1a: quinidine, procainamide, disopyramide
- 1b: lidocaine, phenytoin, mexilitene, tocainide
- 1c: encainide, flecainide, propafenone

Class II: β adrenergic receptor antagonists (examples)
- Propranolol, flecainide, propafenone

Class III: Potassium channel blockers (examples)
- Bretylium, sotalol, amiodarone, ibutilide (not available in United Kingdom)

Class IV: Calcium channel blockers (examples)
- Verapamil, diltiazem, nifedipine

Table 18.2 Rhythm disturbances associated with digoxin intoxication.

- Sinus bradycardia
- Sinoatrial block
- First, second, and third degree atrioventricular block
- Atrial tachycardia (with or without atrioventricular block)
- Accelerated junctional rhythm
- Junctional tachycardia
- Ventricular tachycardia or fibrillation

Table 18.3 Drugs causing prolongation of QT interval.

Amiodarone, astemizole, bepridil, bretylium, cisapride, cocaine, tricyclic antidepressants, cyproheptadine, disopyramide, erythromycin, flecainide, thioridazine, pimozide, ibutilide, itraconazole, ketoconazole, phenothiazines, procainamide, propafenone, quinidine, quinine, sotalol, terfenadine, vasopressin

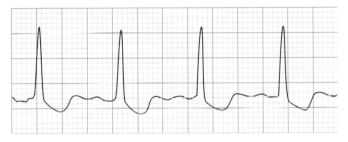

Figure 18.3 Digoxin effect.

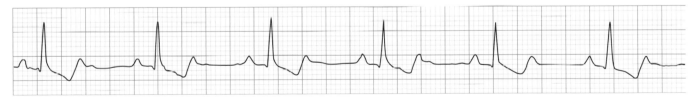

Figure 18.4 Atrial tachycardia with block.

Quinidine-like drugs

The class Ia antiarrhythmic effect is caused by the inhibition of fast sodium channels. Many drugs (for example, disopyramide) share this effect to varying degrees and can share the pro-arrhythmic character of quinidine. Electrocardiographic indicators of toxic effects of quinidine include widening of the QRS complex, prolongation of the QT interval, and atrioventricular nodal blocks. The prolongation of the QT interval predisposes to the development of polymorphic ventricular tachycardia. Slowing of atrial arrhythmia combined with improved atrioventricular conduction (anticholinergic effect) can cause an increase in the ventricular rate response to atrial tachyarrhythmias.

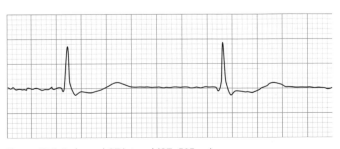

Figure 18.5 Prolonged QT interval (QTc 505 ms).

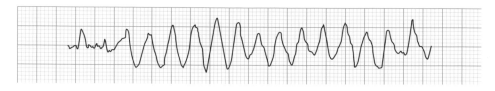

Figure 18.6 Polymorphic ventricular tachycardia in a patient with quinidine intoxication.

Flecainide-like drugs

Flecainide, propafenone, and moracizine can cause bundle branch block. These drugs slow atrial tachycardias and can lead to a paradoxical increase of the ventricular response rate. Monomorphic ventricular tachycardia may also occur.

Congenital heart disease

The electrocardiographic findings associated with congenital lesions of the heart may be subtle, but generally they increase in direct proportion to the severity of the malformation's impact on the patient's physiology. Electrocardiographic abnormalities in children with heart murmurs should increase the clinician's suspicion of a structural lesion. Electrocardiography, however, has been replaced largely by echocardiography for diagnosing and monitoring congenital heart disease. Some congenital lesions are discussed below; others are not included either because they are associated with relatively normal electrocardiograms or because the disease is rare.

Acyanotic lesions

Atrial septal defects

An atrial septal defect results from incomplete closure of the atrial septum in utero. The electrocardiogram may appear relatively normal, with normal P waves in most cases. PR interval prolongation and first degree heart block may occur in up to 20% of cases, but higher grade atrioventricular blocks are uncommon. QRS complexes may show some right ventricular conduction delay denoted by an rsR[1] in V1, but this may also be a normal variant. Associated mitral valve clefts can occur, leading to mitral regurgitation and, if severe, left ventricular hypertrophy. The QRS axis can help to differentiate the two predominant types of atrial septal defect in the following way:

- Ostium primum QRS axis: leftwards (−30° to −90°)
- Ostium secundum QRS axis: rightwards (0 to 180°), with most being more than 100°
- Sinus venosus P wave axis: low atrial pacemaker.

Ventricular septal defects

Ventricular septal defects are the most common cardiac defects at birth. Small ventricular septal defects close spontaneously in 50-70% of cases during childhood. Generally these are not associated with any electrocardiographic abnormalities. As a rule the degree of the electrocardiographic abnormality is directly proportional to the haemodynamic effect on ventricular function. A medium sized ventricular septal defect can exhibit left ventricular hypertrophy and left atrial enlargement. A large ventricular septal

Table 18.4 Differential diagnosis with selected electrocardiographic findings in congenital heart disease.

Axis deviation or hypertrophy
- Superior QRS axis: atrioventricular septal defects, tricuspid atresia
- Left ventricular hypertrophy: aortic stenosis, hypertrophic cardiomyopathy
- Right ventricular hypertrophy: tetralogy of Fallot, severe pulmonary stenosis, secundum atrioventricular septal defect
- Combined ventricular hypertrophy: large ventricular septal defect, atrioventricular septal defect

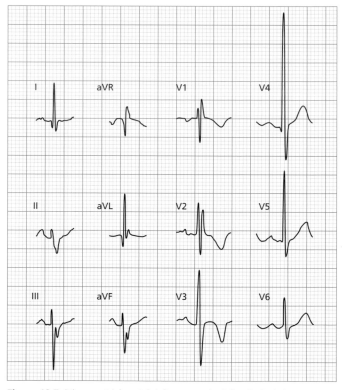

Figure 18.7 Primum atrial septal defect: note the left axis deviation (superior axis).

defect results in biventricular hypertrophy and equiphasic QRS complexes in the mid-precordium known as the Katz-Wachtel phenomenon.

Coarctation of the aorta

Coarctation of the aorta results in left ventricular hypertrophy in 50-60% of asymptomatic children and adults. The strain pattern of lateral T wave inversions is seen in about only 20% of asymptomatic children and adults. ST-T wave abnormalities in the lateral precordial leads are not associated with simple coarctation and

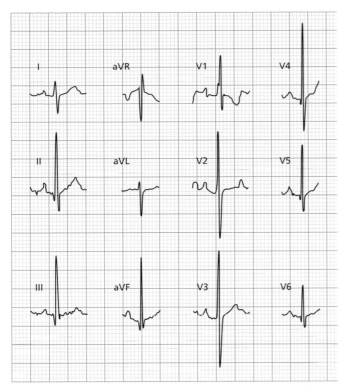

Figure 18.8 Secundum atrial septal defect: note the right axis deviation and dominant R wave in lead V1.

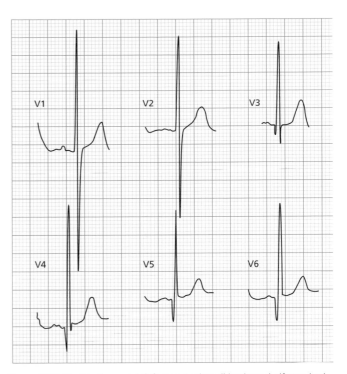

Figure 18.9 Ventricular septal defect: note that all leads are half standard calibration. The biventricular hypertrophy pattern is typical of a ventricular septal defect.

imply additional cardiac disease—for example, left ventricular outflow obstruction. Generally left atrial abnormalities are not seen unless mitral regurgitation develops.

Ebstein's anomaly

Ebstein's anomaly is the downward displacement of the tricuspid valve into the right ventricle causing "atrialisation" of the upper segment of the right ventricle. Tricuspid insufficiency is common, leading to dilation of the right atria, which is indicated by tall peaked P waves in lead II and the anterior leads V1-2. The conduction system itself may be altered by this anomaly, leading to right bundle branch block (complete or incomplete) in 75-80% of patients, a widened QRS complex, or widened PR interval prolongation, or both of the latter. Additionally, there is an association with the Wolff-Parkinson-White syndrome in up to 25% of cases.

Dextrocardia

Dextrocardia is the presence of the heart in the right side of the chest. It can occur alone or in association with situs inversus (complete inversion of the abdominal organs).

Examination of the electrocardiogram in situs inversus will show two obvious abnormalities: loss of the normal precordial R wave progression (prominent right and diminished left lateral precordial forces) and presence of inverted P-QRS-T waves in lead I. If the electrocardiogram has been recorded correctly, and the patient is in sinus rhythm, the presence of an inverted P wave in lead I indicates dextrocardia.

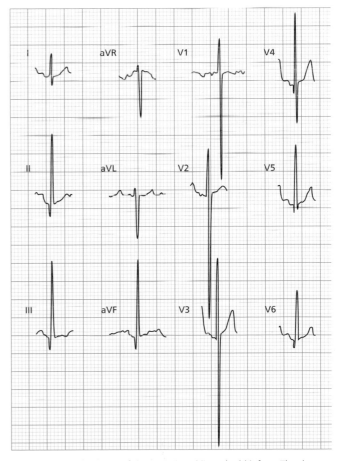

Figure 18.10 Coarctation of the aorta in a 10 week old infant. The deep S wave seen in V1 reflecting striking left ventricular hypertrophy.

Tricuspid atresia

An atrial septal defect must be present to allow for any circulation in the presence of tricuspid atresia. The typical electrocardiographic changes associated with atrial septal defects are seen as well as left axis deviation. Right atrial enlargement occurs and is indicated by tall P waves in leads I, II, and V1. Often there is an associated ventricular septal defect. Occasionally PR interval pro-

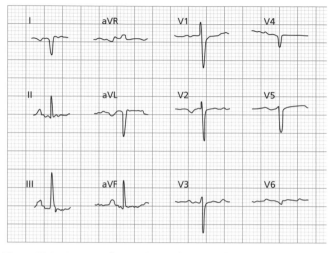

Figure 18.11 Dextrocardia: note inverted P wave in lead I and poor R wave progression.

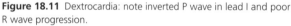

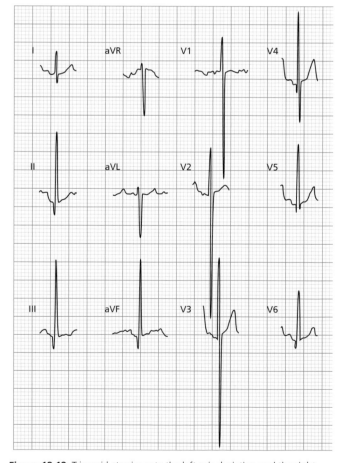

Figure 18.12 Tricuspid atresia: note the left axis deviation and the right atrial enlargement.

longation occurs and a "pseudo pre-excitation" delta wave (not caused by an actual accessory pathway) is seen.

Cyanotic lesions

At birth the normal infant's electrocardiogram will show a right ventricular predominance. Over the first month of life the left ventricle becomes more prominent than the right, and precordial voltage and QRS axis reflect this change. In the cyanotic lesions of the heart, this right sided dominance often persists because there is an increase in pulmonary pressure and resultant hypertrophy of the right ventricle relative to the left.

Tetralogy of Fallot

There are no specific electrocardiographic signs for diagnosing tetralogy of Fallot. Right axis deviation and right ventricular hypertrophy are common, however, so their absence should put the diagnosis of Fallot's tetralogy into question. The presence of a left axis deviation in a patient with a known Fallot's tetralogy suggests a complete atrioventricular canal.

Congenitally corrected transposition of the great arteries

In congenitally corrected transposition of the great arteries, Q waves will be absent in the left precordial leads and prominent in the right. As many as a third of these patients will develop a congenital third degree atrioventricular nodal block.

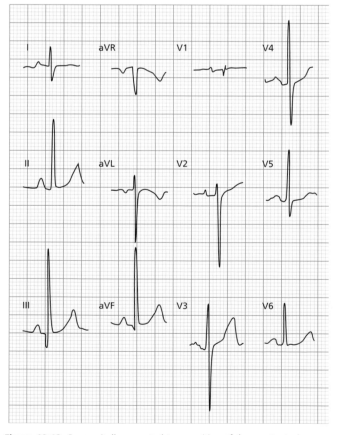

Figure 18.13 Congenitally corrected transposition of the great arteries: note the absence of Q waves in lead 1, V5, and V6, which is characteristic of this lesion.

Self Assessment Quiz

Question 1
A 77 year old female complains of epigastric pain and dizziness. What does the rhythm strip reveal (Lead II)?

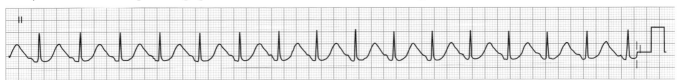

Question 2
An 88 year old man presents with recurrent episodes of dizziness. What is the ECG diagnosis?

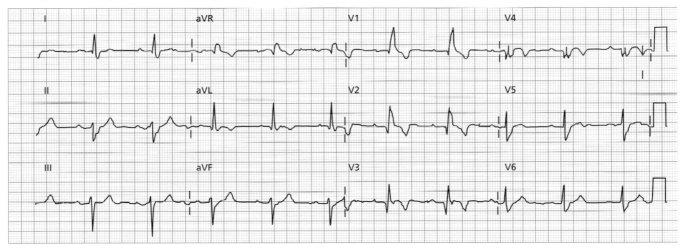

Question 3
A 17 year old woman complains of palpitations and dizziness. What is the ECG diagnosis?

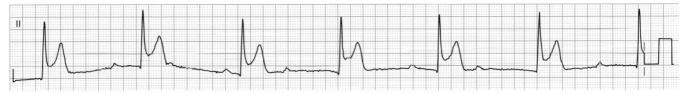

Question 4
What is the diagnosis?

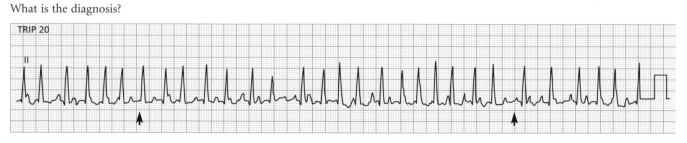

Question 5
A 35 year old man presents with chest pain. What is the ECG diagnosis?

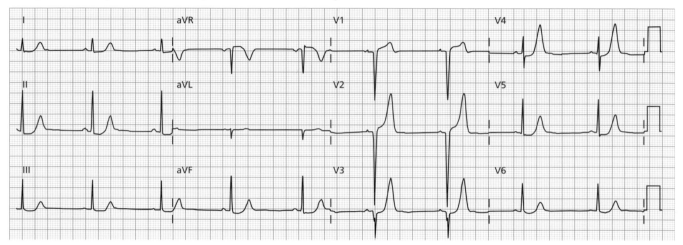

Question 6
What is the ECG diagnosis?

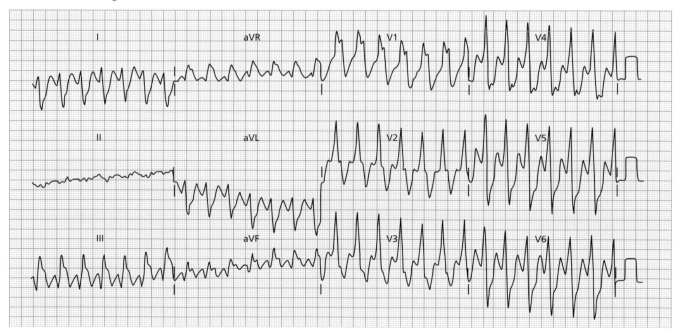

Question 7

What is the ECG diagnosis?

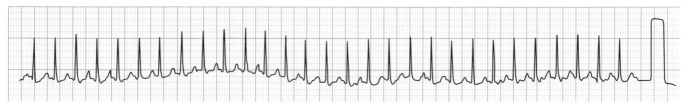

Question 8

What is the ECG diagnosis?

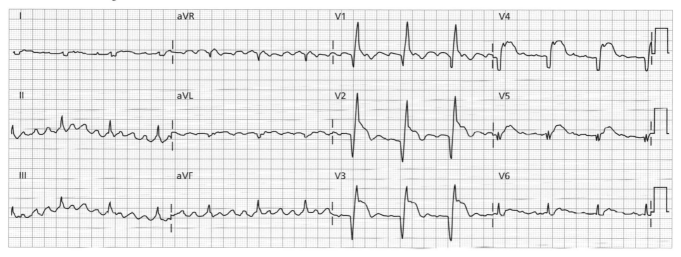

Question 9

What is the rhythm?

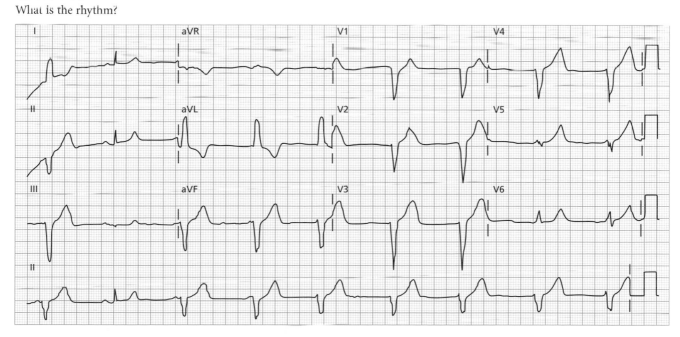

Question 10

An 80 year old man presents with nausea and dizziness. What is the ECG diagnosis?

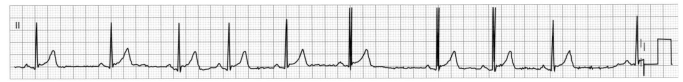

Question 11

What is the rhythm?

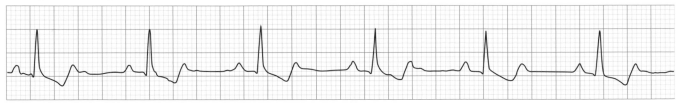

Question 12

What is the rhythm?

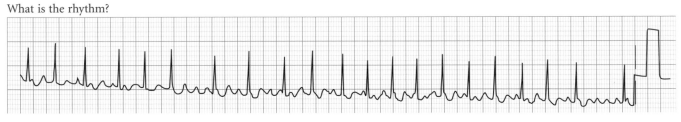

Question 13

What is the rhythm?

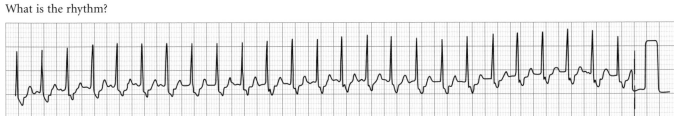

Question 14

An elderly female is found on the floor with a fractured hip. What is the ECG diagnosis?

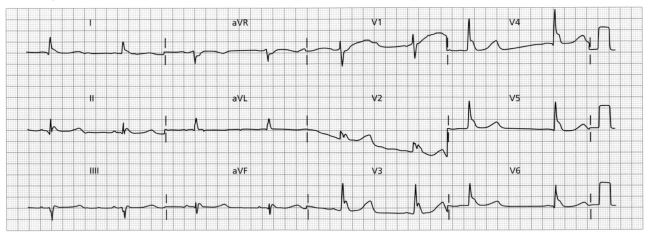

Question 15
A young woman complains of recurrent palpitations. What is the ECG diagnosis?

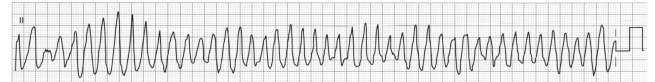

Question 16
A 63 year old man complains of atypical chest pain. What is the diagnosis?

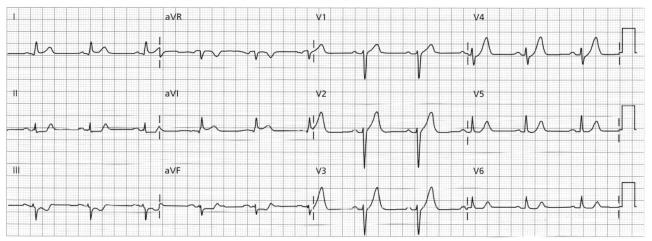

Question 17
A 93 year old woman presents with shortness of breadth. What is the ECG diagnosis?

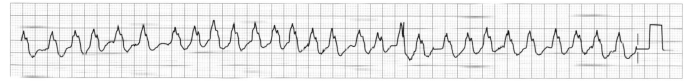

Question 18
A 40 year old man presents with chest pain. What is the ECG diagnosis?

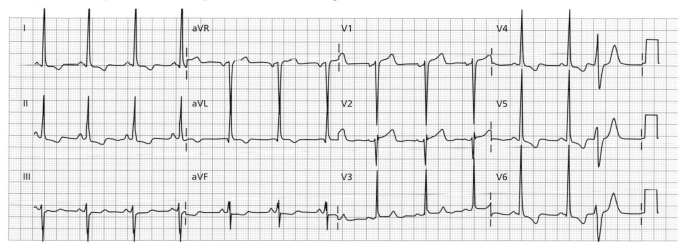

Question 19

A 38 year old man has been feeling generally unwell for several weeks. What is the ECG diagnosis?

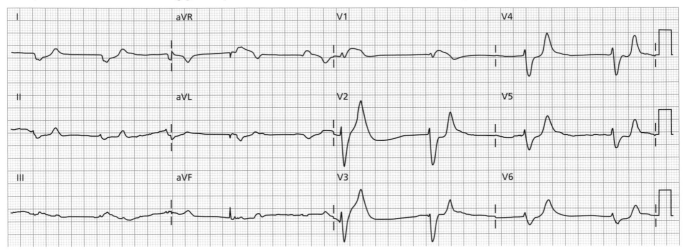

Question 20

An elderly man presents in a collapsed state. What is the rhythm?

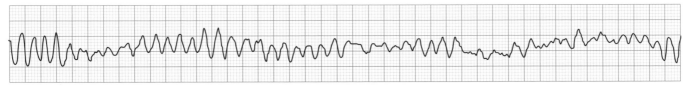

Question 21

A young man complains of chest pain that is worse on palpation. What is the ECG diagnosis?

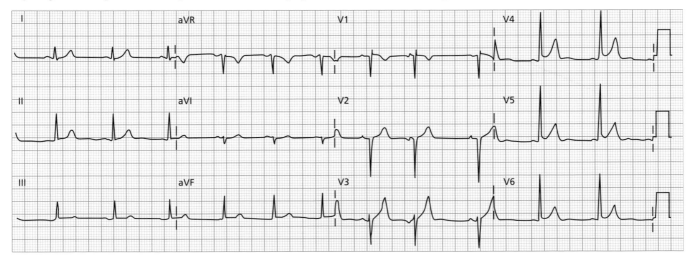

Question 22

A 27 year old man presents with chest pain worse on movement. What is the ECG diagnosis?

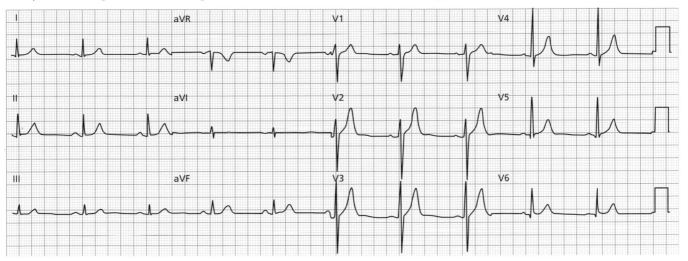

Question 23

A 47 year old woman complains of central chest pain. What is the diagnosis?

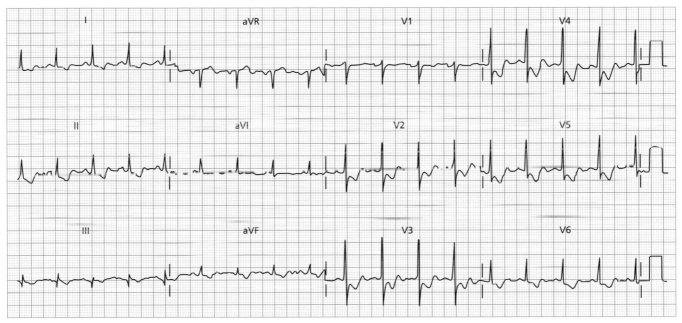

Question 24

A 76 year old woman with hypertension presents with palpitations. What is the ECG diagnosis?

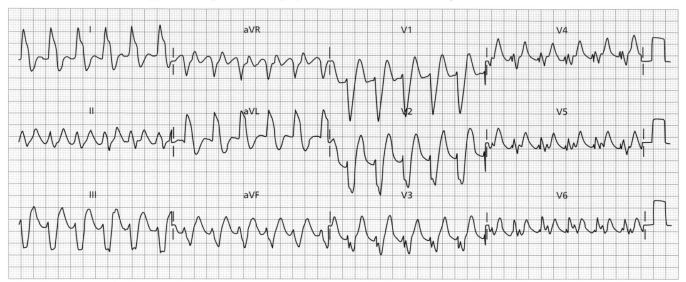

Question 25

A 67 year old man develops chest pain and is hypotensive. What is the ECG diagnosis?

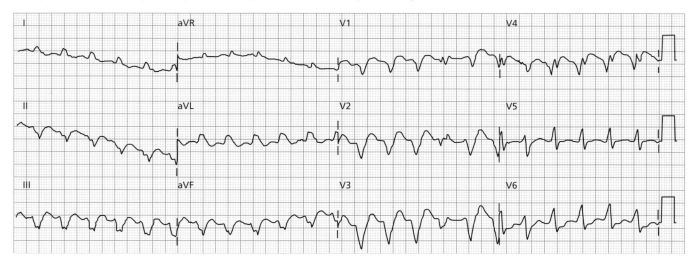

Question 26
A 23 year old man complains of palpitations. What is the ECG diagnosis?

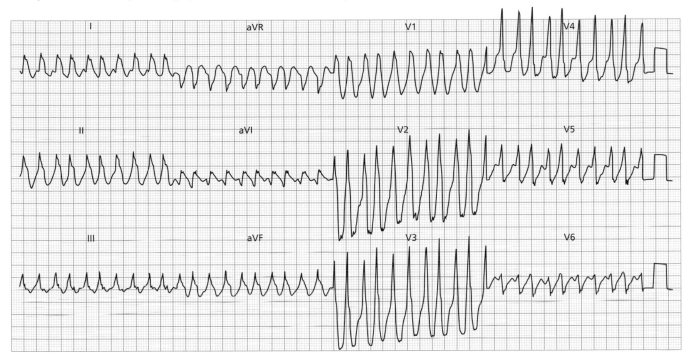

Question 27
A 48 year old man complains of pain on swallowing. What is the ECG diagnosis?

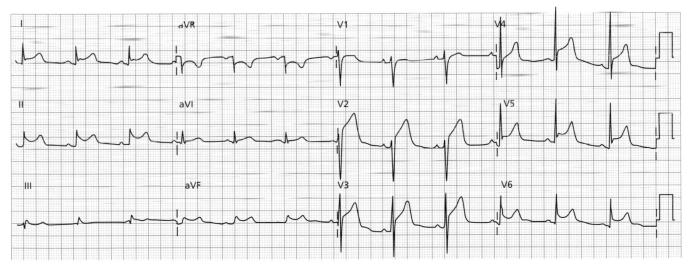

Question 28

A woman complains of central chest pain. What is the diagnosis?

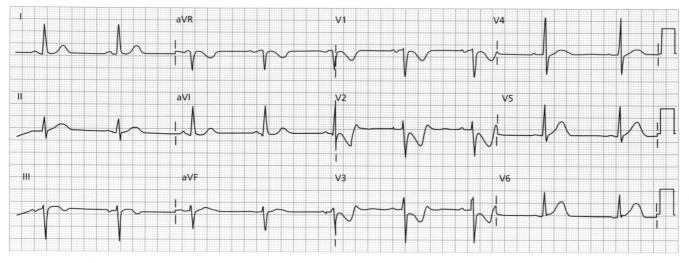

Answers

Answer 1

Third degree heart block and ST segment elevation associated with an inferior myocardial infraction.
(See Chapter 8.)

Answer 2

Trifascicular block. Exhibited by right bundle branch block. Left axis deviation and first degree heart block.

Answer 3

Prolonged QT interval. The QT interval measures 0.56 seconds. The QT interval is greater than 50% of the R-R interval.

Answer 4

Multifocal atrial tachycardia.

Answer 5

Myocardial ischaemia. Peaked T waves in association with widespread ST segment depression.
(See Chapter 10.)

Answer 6

Regular broad complex tachycardia—ventricular tachycardia. The abnormal axis, right bundle branch block pattern and concordance all strongly suggest ventricular tachycardia.

Answer 7

Regular narrow complex tachycardia. The rate and absence of P waves suggest that this rhythm is an atrioventricular nodal re-entry tachycardia (AVNRT).

Answer 8

Anterior myocardial infarction. Right bundle branch block. Atrial flutter.

Answer 9

An idioventricular rhythm. Note the second beat is sinus.
(See Chapter 6.)

Answer 10

Atrial tachycardia with 2:1 block due to digoxin toxicity.

Answer 11

Sinus arrhythmia.

Answer 12

Atrial fibrillation. Note the coarse fibrillation waves.
(See Chapter 4.)

Answer 13

Regular narrow complex tachycardia—atrioventricular re-entry tachycardia (AVRT). The presence of an inverted P wave in the ST segment indicates the presence of an accessory pathway.

Answer 14

Hypothermia. Sinus bradycardia and J waves in the anterior chest leads.

Answer 15

Polymorphic ventricular tachycardia. A fast broad complex tachycardia that is irregular. Note the variable morphology of the QRS complexes. This patient had a prolonged QT interval when in sinus rhythm. Her resting ECG is seen in Question 3.

Answer 16

Evolving anterolateral myocardial infarction. Subtle ST segment elevation is present in lead I, aVL and peaked T waves in the anterior chest leads. Note the reciprocal changes in the inferior leads.

Answer 17

A broad complex tachycardia that is irregular. There is atrial fibrillation with left bundle brand block.

Answer 18

Left ventricular hypertrophy with tall R waves in association with ST segment depression.

Answer 19

Hyperkalaemia. Broad complexes with peaked T waves. Absent P waves.

Answer 20

Ventricular fibrillation.

Answer 21

Benign early repolarisation. There is a notch at the J point in association with ST segment elevation which is most marked in lead V4.

Answer 22

Normal ECG.

Answer 23

A myocardial ischaemic widespread ST depression and T wave inversion.

(See Chapter 3.)

Answer 24

Regular broad complex tachycardia. Default diagnosis is ventricular tachycardia. In this case, however, the correct diagnosis was atrial flutter with rate dependent bundle branch block.

Answer 25

Ventricular tachycardia with left bundle branch pattern. Note the presence of a fusion beat as the fourth complex in leads V1 – V3.

Answer 26

Irregular broad complex tachycardia. Atrial fibrillation in a patient with Wolff-Parkinson-White syndrome. Note the variable morphology of the QRS complexes.

Answer 27

Pericarditis. There is widespread ST segment elevation and, with the exception of aVR, there are no reciprocal changes.

Answer 28

Posterior myocardial infarction.

Index